Doorway Thoughts Editorial Board

Series Editorial Committee

Sharon A. Brangman, MD
Professor of Medicine
Division Chief, Geriatrics
SUNY Upstate Medical University
Syracuse, NY

Marita Grudzen, MHS
Co-Director
Stanford Geriatric Education Center
Stanford University School of Medicine
Stanford, CA

Gwen Yeo, PhD, AGSF
Co-Director
Stanford Geriatric Education Center
Stanford, CA

Contributors

Chapter 1: Introduction
Marita Grudzen, MHS
Co-Director
Stanford Geriatric Education Center
Stanford University School of Medicine
Stanford, CA

Gwen Yeo, PhD, AGSF
Co-Director
Stanford Geriatric Education Center
Stanford, CA

Chapter 2: American Indian Traditions and Theologies
Levanne R. Hendrix, GNP, MSN, PhD
Quality Manager, Extended Care Service,
    Palo Alto VA Health Care System
Asst. Clinical Professor, UCSF School of Nursing
Ethnogeriatric Specialist, Stanford Geriatric
    Education Center
Palo Alto, CA

Father Hank LeBeau (Lakota, Cheyenne River),
    MDiv
Asst. Priest, St. Phillips Episcopal Church
First Nations Ministries
Substance Abuse Counselor, Indian Health Center
    of Santa Clara Valley
San Jose, CA

Chapter 3: Buddhism
Rev. Ronald Y. Nakasone, PhD
Center for Art, Religion, and Education
Core Doctoral Faculty
Graduate Theological Union
Berkeley, CA

Chapter 4: Christianity
Rev. James W. Ellor, PhD
Editor, Journal of Religion, Spirituality and Aging
Director, Center for Gerontological Studies
Professor
School of Social Work
Baylor University
Waco, TX

James P. Oberle, S.S., PhD, STL
Director, Clergy Formation Archdiocese of
    Anchorage Pastor
Our Lady of the Lake
Big Lake, AK

Chapter 5: Hinduism
Vyjeyanthi S. Periyakoil, MD
Clinical Assistant Professor,
Director, Hospice and Palliative Medicine
    Fellowship Program
Stanford University School of Medicine
Palo Alto, CA

Arun S. Rao, MD
Assistant Professor of Medicine
Division of Geriatrics & Gerontology
Weill-Cornell College of Medicine
New York, NY

Pushpendra Sharma, MD
Internal Medicine, Geriatrics
The Jewish Home & Hospital Lifecare System
New York, NY

Chapter 6: Islam
Kamyar M. Hedayat, MD, FAAP
Attending, Critical Care
Department of Pediatrics
Advocate Lutheran Children's Hospital
Chicago, IL

Dr. Ahmed Nezar Kobeisy
Muslim Chaplain & Adjunct Faculty
Syracuse University
Le Moyne College and Hartford Seminary
Syracuse, NY

Doha Raik Hamza
Muslim Volunteer Coordinator (2003–2007)
Spiritual Care Services at Stanford Hospital
Alexandria, Egypt

Chapter 7: Judaism

Chaplain Bruce Feldstein, MD
Spiritual Care Service, Stanford Hospital & Clinics
Director, The Jewish Chaplaincy at Stanford
  University Medical Center
Adjunct Clinical Professor, Center for Education
  in Family and Community Medicine, Stanford
  University School of Medicine
Stanford, CA

Chaplain D'vorah Rose, RN, MA
Spiritual Care Service, Stanford Hospital & Clinics
Associate Chaplain, The Jewish Chaplaincy at
  Stanford University Medical Center
Stanford, CA

Carol Hutner-Winograd, MD
Associate Professor of Medicine and Human
  Biology, Emerita
Stanford University
Stanford, CA

Chapter 8: Shamanism

Pa Lor
Hmong Shaman
Stockton, CA

Marilyn Mochel, RN
Cultural Competence Training Consultant
Merced, CA

Chapter 9: Sikhism

Upinder Singh, MD, CMD, AGSF, FACP
Clinical Associate Professor
University of Nevada School of Medicine
Chief of Geriatics
SMA, Sierra Health Services
Las Vegas, NV

Chapter 10: Confucianism and Daoism

Catherine Eng, MD, FACP
Clinical Professor of Medicine, UCSF
Medical Director, On Lok Senior Health Services
San Francisco, CA

Edmond Yee, C. Phil., PhD
Professor of Asian Studies
Pacific Lutheran Theological Seminary
Core Doctoral Faculty
Graduate Theological Union
Berkeley, CA

Medical Editor

Susan E. Aiello, DVM, ELS
WordsWorld Consulting
Dayton, OH

Doorway Thoughts: Cross-Cultural Health Care for Older Adults, Volume 1:

Introduction to Cross-Cultural Health Care for Older Adults

Older American Indians and Alaska Natives

Older Hispanic Americans

Older African Americans

Older Vietnamese Americans

Older Asian Indian Americans

Older Japanese Americans

Older Chinese Americans

(Available from the publisher: ISBN-10: 0-7637-3338-5, paperback)

Doorway Thoughts: Cross-Cultural Health Care for Older Adults, Volume 2:

Older Arab Americans

Older Cambodian Americans

Older Filipino Americans

Older Haitian Americans

Older Korean Americans

Older Pakistani Americans

Older Portuguese Americans

Older Russian-Speaking Americans

(Available from the publisher: ISBN-10: 0-7637-4355-0, paperback)

To order, call 1-800-832-0034 or visit www.jbpub.com.

CONTENTS

Acknowledgments

The editorial committee wishes to thank everyone involved in the development of this third and final volume of *Doorway Thoughts*: the authors, who gave so generously of their time and experience in writing each chapter; the Ethnogeriatrics Committee of the American Geriatrics Society (AGS), whose hard work and dedication paved our way; the AGS Board of Directors, committee chairs, and members for their invaluable comments and suggestions; our medical editor, Susan E. Aiello, DVM, ELS; and Christine Campanelli and the AGS staff, who have been essential to the success of this volume.

Editorial Committee:
Sharon Brangman, MD, FACP, AGSF
Marita Grudzen, MHS
Cynthia X. Pan, MD, AGSF, FACP
Gwen Yeo, PhD

CHAPTER I

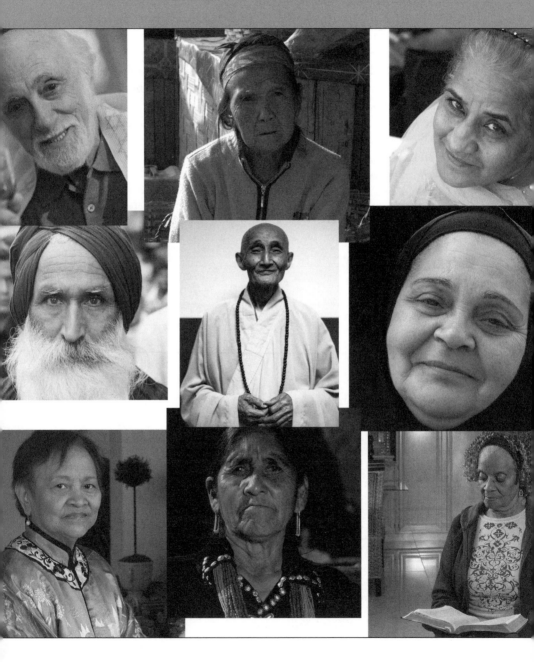

Introduction

In spite of the growing recognition that faith, religious affiliation, and religious participation are important variables in health and outcomes of health interventions, physicians and other health care professionals in the United States receive little formal training in dealing with diverse spiritual and religious issues related to health. "Spirituality is the way you find meaning, hope, and comfort and inner peace in one's life. Many people find spirituality through religion. Some find it through music, art or a connection with nature. Others find it in their values and principles" (American Academy of Family Physicians). Religion is "a more formal system that provides meaning to life through a common set of beliefs, rituals and practices. It provides the structure for spiritual beliefs for most people" (King). The Joint Commission on Accreditation of Healthcare Organizations requires that both spiritual and cultural assessments be performed and integrated into care plans.

Being able to respond to spiritual concerns of patients and their families in the context of chronic or terminal illness is particularly important for older adults, but the complex array of religions and faith communities associated with the rapidly increasing diversity of cultural backgrounds of patients makes appropriate response by health care providers difficult.

This volume is the third in the series of *Doorway Thoughts: Cross-cultural Health Care for Older Adults,* developed by the Ethnogeriatrics Committee of the American Geriatrics Society. The series is designed to better prepare geriatric and gerontologic providers of all disciplines to give culturally competent care when they open the door to see an older patient from one of the dozens of culturally diverse backgrounds in the United States. The committee recognized that, in addition to the discussions of the 15 ethnic backgrounds in Volumes I and II of *Doorway Thoughts,* providers should have information and resources about the wide variety of religious and spiritual needs that diverse older adults may bring to the health care encounter.

Effect of Religion and Spirituality on Health

Building on extensive literature that indicates that individuals who describe themselves as religious are more likely to have better health indicators, Koenig and colleagues found that among 838 older hospitalized patients, religiousness and spirituality consistently predicted greater social support, fewer depressive symptoms, better cognitive and physical function, less severe illness and co-morbidity, and better general health. Those who categorized themselves as neither spiritual nor religious tended to have worse self- and observer-rated health and greater medical comorbidity. When illness strikes, religion and spirituality can be important for coping, which emphasizes the necessity for providers to be skilled in helping older patients access spiritual resources to provide support and facilitate healing.

When illness strikes, religion and spirituality can be important for coping, which emphasizes the necessity for providers to be skilled in helping older patients access spiritual resources to provide support and facilitate healing.

Approach to the Patient

As all the authors in the following chapters emphasize, within every religious community there is a wide range of commitment to, and participation in, the tenets and activities of every faith. For providers to provide effective spiritual support, they must make no *a priori* assumptions about the degree to which older people and their families need the support of representatives of their faith communities. Identifying one's religion or religious affiliation on hospital or clinical records may or may not imply being comfortable with the presence of clergy or chaplains.

Taking a brief spiritual history is an important first step. As health care providers enter into this process, we need to be aware of our own cultural and spiritual beliefs and how they affect our attitudes and practice. Two models, FICA and HOPE, explore patients' sources of hope, strength, and meaning, including spirituality and religion. We recommend combining FICA and HOPE in the following way:

- Choose one of the following opening phrases:
  "For some people, their spiritual or religious beliefs are an important source of comfort and strength in dealing with illness and suffering. Is this true for you?"
  "What has given you strength during difficult times in the past?"
  "We know that one's spiritual and religious beliefs can affect their health…"

- **F**aith/Beliefs:
  Do you consider yourself spiritual or religious?
  What is your faith or belief?
  What things do you believe in that give meaning to your life?

- **I**mportance/Influence:
  How have your beliefs influenced your behaviors during this illness?
  What role do your beliefs play in regaining your health?

- **C**ommunity:
  Are you a part of a spiritual or religious community?
  Is there a person or group of people you really love or who are really important to you?

- **A**ddress:
  How would you like me as your physician (or other health care provider) to address these issues in your care and in this setting?

With use of the FICA assessment tool, the patient or family can identify the spiritual leader, companion, or minister (if there is one) who could assist with the spiritual needs or concerns of the patient. When that information is not available, typically the hospital chaplaincy or pastoral care program can assist for inpatients. Many of these spiritual care programs have spiritual care volunteers from different cultural and religious traditions. The cultural representative of a faith community can be critical in discerning the significance of a particular spiritual issue.

> *The cultural representative of a faith community can be critical in discerning the significance of a particular spiritual issue.*

Spiritual Support for the Decision-Making Process

When confronted by the need to make life-altering decisions about whether or not to undergo major treatments, many older adults and their families find the assistance of religious counselors or chaplains very helpful. This becomes even more salient in the context of very serious or terminal illness. To provide effective geriatric care at those critical times, providers need to be able to comfortably inquire about the patient's or the family's preference for including a representative from their faith community or chaplain on the health care team (and then have the skills to integrate that person if one is requested). This can be especially important when questions of do-not-resuscitate orders are being considered.

Incorporating Spiritual Advisors into the Health Care Team

Knowing where to find individuals who can take on the role of spiritual adviser in the health care setting is the first challenge in accommodating older patients' preferences for including such advisers. Chaplains trained in Clinical Pastoral Education are trained to minister to diverse spiritual needs. The chaplains are also typically aware of the diversity of religious backgrounds that older adults bring to the health care setting. When they are not aware of religious leaders of a particular tradition, they try to identify those resources for the patient. On the other hand, sometimes when older patients become ill and are not at peace with the situation, they can become disillusioned or angry at their spiritual or religious representative, and they might benefit more from a health care chaplain who is a bit more removed from their particular faith.

Patients and families have their own experiences, cultural and spiritual values, and beliefs that may only resonate with a cultural or spiritual representative who can amplify their voice.

When a patient is experiencing spiritual distress and/or confusion or conflict in health care decision making, it is critical to include spiritual care and cultural (when appropriate) resources in any team conferences. Spiritual care experts can contribute to the care process whether or not the older patient accepts direct spiritual interventions. The identified spiritual adviser could also be helpful if invited to attend meetings with older patients and/or family members around important decision points. These encounters include many cultural belief systems and practices. For health professionals, there is the hospital culture, the professional cultures represented, the spiritual cultures, and the many personal values that operate in that context. Patients and families have their own experiences, cultural and spiritual values, and beliefs that may only resonate with a cultural or spiritual representative who can amplify their voice. Sometimes, it is the only way the needs or choices of the patient and family can be understood.

Marita Grudzen
Gwen Yeo

References

American Academy of Family Physicians. Spirituality and Health Information handout for patients, 2001. Available at: http://familydoctor.org/650.xml (accessed August 2005).

Anandarajah GG, Hight E. Spirituality and medical practice: using the HOPE questions as a practical tool for spiritual assessment. *Am Fam Physician* 2001;65(1):81–88.

Joint Commission on Accreditation of Healthcare Organizations. Implementation section of the 1996 standards for hospitals by JCAHO. Oakbrook Terrace, IL: Joint Commission on Accreditation of Healthcare Organizations; 1996.

King DE. *Faith, Spirituality and Medicine; Toward the Making of the Healing Practitioner.* New York: Haworth Press; 2000.

Koenig H, George L, Titus P. Religion, spirituality, and health in medically ill hospitalized older patients. *J Am Ger Soc* 2004;52:554–562.

Puchalski CM, Romer AL. Taking a spiritual history allows clinicians to understand patients more fully. *J Palliat Med* 2000;3(1):129–137.

CHAPTER 2

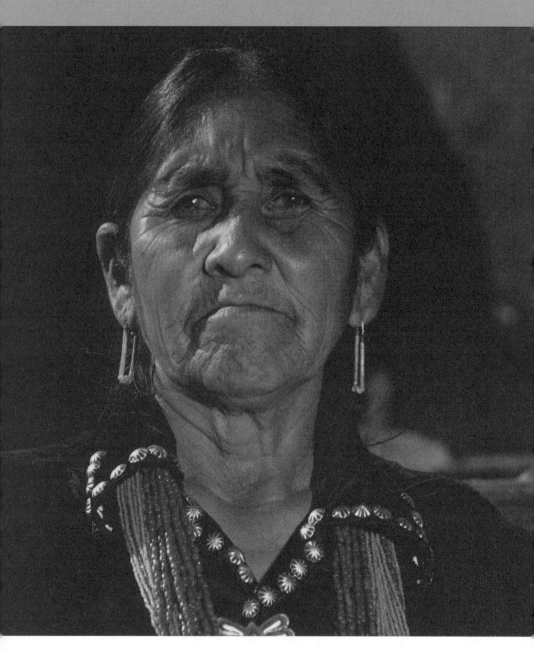

American Indian Traditions and Theologies

"We should understand well that all things are the works of the Great Spirit. We should know that He is within all things: the trees, the grasses, the rivers, the mountains, and all the four-legged animals, and the winged peoples; and even more important, we should understand that He is also above all these things and peoples. When we do understand all this deeply in our hearts, then we will fear, and love, and know the Great Spirit, and then we will be and act and live as He intends."

— BLACK ELK (OGLALA SIOUX)

Manderson SD. Preface to *The Sacred Pipe: Black Elk's Account of the Seven Rites of the Oglala Sioux*. Recorded and edited by Joseph Epes Brown. Norman, OK: University of Oklahoma Press. 1959, 1989. pp xix-xx.

History

There is no single "American Indian religion." There are over 550 federally recognized Indian Nations (tribes), and some 300 different languages. American Indian peoples, their cultures, and theologies are heterogeneous and diverse.

American Indian peoples, their cultures, and theologies are heterogeneous and diverse.

Before European domination, American Indian nations had well-developed and practiced theologies, including holy lands and sacred sites, spiritual systems of belief and practice, holy men and women who assisted in maintaining the connection between the people and God (the Creator of all things, the Great Mystery, Great Spirit), and prophets who appeared to the people at various times in indigenous history. The sacred is considered as a noun (rather than an adjective) and was present in North America long before the White man set foot on this land. Many historical and contemporary American Indians feel that it was a measure of the White man's theology of conquest and violence, as well as greed for the land, that promoted Christian missionizing at the cost of native theologies. In the late 19th and early 20th centuries, many Christian religious groups rigidly condemned Indian theologies as "heathen" and worthless, and all traditional Indian religious practices were outlawed. These included important religious ceremonies widely practiced in many tribes, such as the Sun Dance, the Ghost Dance, and the Peyote ceremony, even though the latter two were based on belief systems that incorporated some Christian aspects. Despite these attacks, the concepts inherent in First Nations theology have survived. Today, First Nations ceremonies and traditions are being sought out by disillusioned non-Indians and contemporary Indians alike. It may be said that American Indian theologies and ideologies are providing a "conscience" for the Americas today, in that the "sacred," which values preservation of the environment, was already here and not imported by colonization.

Most traditional Indian socialization focused on the community rather than on the individual, whereby the family functions within the traditions of the clan.

Most traditional Indian socialization focused on the community rather than on the individual, whereby the family functions within the traditions of the clan. In urban areas, a philosophy of "pan-Indianism" operates to strengthen the Indian community, as there are representatives from many different nations and traditions.

Older Indian people tend to be cared for within the Indian community by friends and families. Nursing home admission is infrequent, and use of long-term care services is very low. Reasons include 1) lack of knowledge of how to access services; 2) complexity of the Indian health care system, especially when combined with Medicare and Medicaid eligibility requirements; 3) distrust of the Western medical system, the federal government, and health care providers; and 4) lack of comfort with service providers.

First Nations Theologies and Christianity

"Conversion" to Christianity by many American Indians was facilitated by the inclusive nature of Indian thinking, in that new practices and rituals could be added to the existing culture for community enhancement. Many Indian Nations, in the face of devastating losses through disease epidemics and by the relentless invasion of White people into Indian lands, came to believe that the White man's God must be more powerful than the Indian ways, and added Christian beliefs to their lives.

Similarities between American Indian theologies and Christian heritage made it easier for Indians to accept the missionaries' message. This included the fact that most Indian theologies and oral histories had prophets and mystics that were sent by the Great Spirit (God) to help the people and teach them good ways (eg, Buffalo Calf Woman) from time to time, as the Christians had Jesus. A definite difference, however, seems to be the concept of a vertical hierarchy to obtain access to God, as taught by Christian missionaries, versus a circular theology including man, nature, fellow man, and God.

"Conversion" to Christianity by many American Indians was facilitated by the inclusive nature of Indian thinking, in that new practices and rituals could be added to the existing culture for community enhancement.

Many American Indian people are second- or third-generation Christians because of training received in the missionary boarding schools. Geographic area of origin is important in that Christian missionaries divided reservation and tribal lands into territories, so as not to "compete for converts." Therefore, the Christian denomination of American Indian people may be geographically determined, and it is likely to be the religion of preference for spiritual support in times of need or illness. In addition, some older American Indian people are turning more to Christian teachings for support as the spiritual advisers and medicine people with traditional knowledge on their home reservations die out.

Just as Christian beliefs are frequently superimposed on the centuries-old Indian theologies, in many communities some traditional Indian rituals and ceremonies are integrated into Christian services. That could include, for example, honoring the Four Sacred Directions as well as the Holy Trinity, and using traditional chants as well as organ music.

Today, there are also controversies within the American Indian Christian theological community based on a variety of issues such as the fact that many Indian theologies come from a different starting place (ie, creation rather than salvation) and that Indian oral history stories are as valid as those in the Bible.

Common Elements in Indian Traditions
Despite the diverse nature of Indian traditions, there are a few commonalities that may be helpful.

- "Sacred" is used as a noun rather than an adjective and is a part of everyday life.

Most Indian theologies include the relationship among God (Creator), nature, self, and others. This relationship may be represented by a circle with you, me, nature, relatives, community, creatures and "all that is" interconnected.

- Most Indian theologies include the relationship among God (Creator), nature, self, and others. This relationship may be represented by a circle with you, me, nature, relatives, community, creatures and "all that is" interconnected. God/Creator is at the center and is present in all things. The Great Mystery or Holy Spirit is the "glue" that connects everything.

- Ceremonies, objects, rituals, and sacred sites are generally protected within the Indian communities, both by tradition and as a result of the federal government making the practice of Indian religion illegal during the 20th century and of the usurping of ceremonies by unscrupulous practitioners for money.

- *All* veterans are especially honored, in the warrior tradition, of having fought to defend Indian land—"The honor of one is the honor of all."

- There is a general belief that there is something after death, which often includes being reunited with relatives who have previously died. Extended family members were all that American Indian people had for support, and it is not uncommon for those getting ready to "cross over to the next world" to be "visited" by relatives who have died.

- Accumulation of possessions is not a cultural value. Honor and social standing is gained by giving away possessions and taking care of the women, children, and old ones.

- Intergenerational trauma and grief is considered in a spiritual context as the ability to survive a holocaust, and as being "the strength of our people." Forgiveness may be "sharing the goodness" of overcoming "hate" and anger.

- "Old ones" are respected and honored as possessing of wisdom, life experience, and traditional cultural knowledge.

- In many American Indian traditions, physical health is considered to be intimately related to spiritual health, and "illness" may be seen as an imbalance. Healing ceremonies can be performed by a medicine man or woman and involve religious rituals. Sweat lodges are sometimes used as purification rituals for healing as well. Medicine and healing are considered a sacred work.

When asked to comment on current spiritual beliefs and practices, urban elders from the Plains, Southwest, and California tribes related stories of the teaching of Indian ways by grandparents or tribal elders in their youth, and the addition of Christianity later in life.

In many American Indian traditions, physical health is considered to be intimately related to spiritual health, and "illness" may be seen as an imbalance.

Spiritual Support

Learning about the people health providers work with is key to providing appropriate spiritual support. Rev. LeBeau recommends an assessment through conversation and uses four general groupings: 1) full-blood/traditional, 2) full-blood/nontraditional, 3) mixed-blood/traditional, and 4) mixed-blood/nontraditional. Diverse practices exist within these groups and can include the practice of only traditional religion (full- or mixed-blood), the beliefs and practices from both Indian theology and Christianity, or a complete conversion to the White man's Christianity with denial of Indian Ways. Therefore it is essential to evaluate the perspective of the individual patient to access supportive services if desired.

If supportive services in a health care setting are desired by an elder with traditional beliefs, these could include bringing in a spiritual adviser from the American Indian community, finding a medicine person from the elder's home (reservation) community to provide healing rituals, supporting the family's arrangement to transport the elder to the home community to participate in a healing ceremony, and/or helping to locate and provide sweet grass and sage or other objects that provide comfort and promote healing in a traditional framework.

Role of the Spiritual Advisor

The goal of spiritual support with an American Indian person is to identify that person's belief (or lack of belief) in "creatorship" and then to follow that path. The basic message is the same in Christianity and Indian theology—surrender and forgiveness lead to transformation, and "before

The goal of spiritual support with an American Indian person is to identify that person's belief (or lack of belief) in "creatorship" and then to follow that path.

anything we need to humble ourselves." Humility is an abiding cultural value for the Indian person.

For example, an angry Indian man attends a mandatory alcohol avoidance group. He enters the room stating that he doesn't want to hear "any God/Jesus stuff." Is he angry about being Indian? About racism? Is he angry at God? Does he believe? Has he had a bad life? (The goal is to assist this man, if possible, to recognize his relationship with a creator—to establish a creatorship and eventual acceptance of who he is.)

Rev. LeBeau suggests an indirect approach in asking about his family (eg, Where did your mother come from? Your father?) *and* starting with a brief self-disclosure and empathy for his situation. Then proceed to talk about the Holy Spirit indirectly by discussing the native cultural value of "all my relations," and asking the question, "What is the glue that holds 'all my relations' together?" The answer involves "the Great Mystery" (the Holy Spirit) and may lead to the man's recognition of his own creatorship belief. This approach includes both Christian and traditional belief systems and can go either way in spiritual support depending on the individual's preferences.

End-of-Life Care

End-of-life spiritual support for First Nations people involves assessment of religious preference as well as eventual acceptance of their fate, who they are, and where they are going to go.

End-of-life spiritual support for First Nations people involves assessment of religious preference as well as eventual acceptance of their fate, who they are, and where they are going to go. Talking about death is considered taboo in one large Southwestern nation, and it is frowned on in other traditions because of the belief that doing so may make it happen. Advance directives and do-not-resuscitate orders are not used very often.

Care of the body after death may be ritually prescribed, as well as care of surgically removed body parts, and should be thoroughly explored with the patient/family if appropriate, using an indirect approach. Some traditions do not allow touching of the body, and the deceased's possessions are not kept by the family.

End Thoughts

First Nations theology has been historically dismissed, or labeled as "Native American wisdom," "mythology," or "spirituality," rather than as theology. In the earliest published works by American Indians until today, American Indian material has a consistent theological content and is not merely romanticized legend. First Nations theologies are living, breathing, evolving theologies, used every day by First Nations people as they revisit the sacred within themselves.

| CASE STUDY **1** | **Sharing Prayer and the Bible with Other Patients** |

Objectives
1. Explain how cultural beliefs of the Lakota Sioux might contribute to apparent fearfulness or anxiety.
2. Discuss the benefit of continued prayer in nursing facilities for American Indian patients with mental health conditions.

Mrs. H. has advanced Alzheimer's disease and entered a skilled nursing facility in an urban setting 2 months ago after her family could no longer care for her safety at their home.

Mrs. H. is full-blood Lakota Sioux, and although she knows her Indian language she does not speak it because, like other elders of her generation, she was punished in boarding school for speaking her language. She learned to "be a proud Indian" by being silent and careful because "there are many enemies, and the enemy is always around" (in her lifetime, "the enemy" often turned out to be non-Indians). In her later years, this cultural teaching for survival contributed to an escalation of paranoid ideation and fearfulness. A major component of Mrs. H.'s fearfulness was that some of her relatives would not be able to join her in the next world (traditional belief system) because they were living in a careless way and would have to bear the consequences. Her Pentecostal Christian beliefs dictated that her relatives would have to accept Christ to be saved. These fears contributed to her lifelong anxiety and stress, and in later years, fears of "being left alone."

The staff at the convalescent center learned from the family that Mrs. H. spent most of her life helping others in her community through sharing of herself and whatever money or food she had. Many years ago, she converted from the Episcopalian Church of her family and childhood to the Pentecostal faith, and her love for Jesus was a guiding force in her life.

Mrs. H. was well known in her community for providing very long prayers when asked. She continued her tradition of providing very long oral prayers in the convalescent home, often repeating herself and losing her words, but the staff came to understand that this was Mrs. H.'s way of continuing to give to her community and the people around her, as she had always done. It was uplifting for her.

As her disease progressed and she was no longer able to read, she continued to quote scripture, and the staff helped her to hold her Bible as if she were reading it. Her Bible was a symbol of her abiding faith and the journey that she was taking with Jesus Christ; it was a great comfort to her in her times of fearfulness, and she kept her Bible close to her until her death.

Question:

1. How can health care personnel facilitate patients' ability to continue spiritual or religious practices?

| CASE STUDY **2** | **I Can't Eat with That in Here!** |

Objective

1. Consider how culturally taboo items in patients' environments can have an impact on their well-being.

Mr. N. (Navajo or Diné) died of renal cancer in a hospice in an urban setting. About 2 months before Mr. N. was admitted to hospice, his family took him back to Indian country. There, he was seen by a Crystal Gazer (traditional diagnostician) and a Hand Trembler (determines which ceremony is appropriate for a diagnosed problem). "Navajo Way" and "Lightening Way" ceremonies were performed by a Singer. During the ceremony, Mr. N. was told that water, "squiggly things," and fish were taboo for him, and he was given a potion that he was to take by mouth.

When Mr. N. was admitted to the hospice, he was assessed as having culturally specific care needs, and the staff set about finding ways to support him and his family spiritually, physically, and emotionally. Mr. N.'s sister-in-law became the spokesperson for the family, and she was asked for information about Navajo traditions and the family's preferences. "Death" was not spoken of directly, based on this information, and the staff felt that further questions at this time would be intrusive and insensitive. (The clinical nurse specialist later asserted that staff may not need to know each tradition, but that there *are* traditions and that they will be different for each family.)

Mr. N. developed a problem with food intake, and a dietician was called. After extensive evaluation and talking with the family, it was found that the wallpaper border in the room contained "trout" in the pattern, and Mr. N. was literally surrounded by taboo elements. The patient was moved as soon as the situation was understood. The staff did not dismiss Mr. N.'s nutritional problem as an expectation of hospice care but continued to evaluate contributing cultural factors that might be alleviated to ensure his quality of care.

Question:

1. How could health care personnel have improved their awareness of Mr. N.'s cultural beliefs in regards to his nutritional intake sooner?

Reprinted with permission. Hendrix LR. Cultural support in health care: the older urban American Indian of the San Francisco bay area. Dissertation. The Union Institute and University, Cincinnati, OH; 1999.

Levanne R. Hendrix, GNP, MSN, PhD
Reverend Hank Swift-Cloud LeBeau, (Lakota) Mdiv

References

Cross A. (Hidatsa). Working with American Indian elders in the city: reflections of an American Indian social worker. In: Yeo G, Gallagher-Thompson D (eds). *Ethnicity and the Dementias* (Chap 15). Washington DC: Taylor & Francis; 1996.

Deloria V Jr, Lytle CM. *American Indians, American Justice*. Austin: University of Texas Press; 1983.

Dorris M. *Paper Trail*. New York: Harper Collins; 1994.

Eastman CA. *The Soul of an Indian*, 1911. Available at: http://www.sacred-texts.com/nam/eassoul.htm.

Finke B, Henderson JN, McCabe M. Older American Indians and Alaska Natives. In: Adler R, Kamel HK (eds). *Doorway Thoughts: Cross-cultural Health Care for Older Adults*. Ethnogeriatrics Committee of the American Geriatrics Society. Sudbury, MA: Jones & Bartlett; 2004.

Hendrix LR. Cultural support in health care: the older urban American Indian of the San Francisco Bay Area. Dissertation. The Union Institute and University, Cincinnati, OH; 1999.

Hendrix LR. Health and health care of American Indian and Alaska Native elders. In: Yeo G (ed). *Ethnic Specific Modules of the Curriculum in Ethnogeriatrics*. Rockville, MD: Bureau of Health Professions, HRSA, US DHHS; 2001. Available at: www.stanford.edu/group/ethnoger.

Hendrix LR. Urban American Indian elders: attitudes and experiences concerning spiritual practices and resources, pain management, and herbal remedies. Paper presented at the 13th Annual Indian Health Service Research Conference, Albuquerque, NM; 2001.

Hendrix LR. Revisiting sacred ways: spiritual support and native American theologies for the health care provider. SGEC Working Paper #16. Stanford, CA: Stanford Geriatric Education Center; 2003.

Hurtado AL. *Indian Survival on the California Frontier*. New Haven, CT: Yale University Press; 1998.

Jackson YM, Manson S, Allery A. Home and community-based long-term care in American Indian and Alaska Native communities. Executive Summary. Washington, DC: Administration on Aging, US DHHS; Native Elder Health Care Resource Center, University of Colorado; National Resource Center on Native American Aging, University of North Dakota. December 1996.

Manson SM. Provider assumptions about long-term care in American Indian communities. *Gerontologist* 1989;29(3):355–358.

Nabakov P (ed). *Native American Testimony: a Chronicle of Indian-White Relations from Prophecy to the Present*. New York: Penguin Books; 1991:1492–1992.

Additional Resources

Indian Health Service, Eldercare Initiative
    Zuni PHS Hospital, PO Box 467, Zuni, NM 87327
    www.ihs.gov/MedicalPrograms/elderCare/index.asp
Recovery Ministries of the Episcopal Church, Inc.
    38439 5th Avenue, #2705, Zephyrhills, FL 33542
    Toll free: 866-306-1542
National Indian Council on Aging, Inc.
    10501 Montgomery Blvd., Suite 210, Albuquerque, NM 87111
    Phone: 505-292-2001; Fax: 505-292-1922
    http://www.nicoa.org
Native Web: http://www.nativeweb.org
Sacred Texts of Native American Religion: http://www.sacred-texts.com/nam/htm

CHAPTER 3

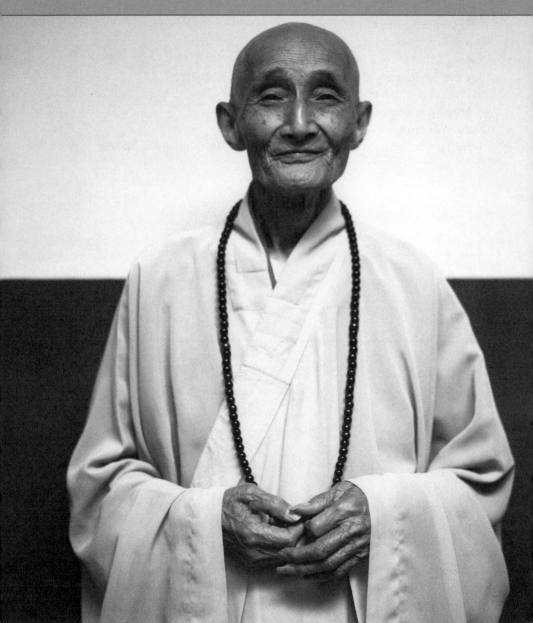

Buddhism

The medical professional caring for a Buddhist devotee may find it helpful to determine whether the patient is of Theravāda or Mahāyāna persuasion, the two Buddhist living traditions. It may also be beneficial to understand the layers of indigenous folk and other beliefs that color the patient's imagination of his or her faith, especially karma, and the patient's degree of acculturation to America and its medical system.

Note: In light of case studies, the description of Buddhist thought and culture in this chapter is partial to the Theravāda Lao-Thai and Mahāyāna Japanese Pure Land Buddhist experiences.

Buddhism in America

Immigrants and refugees from Asia have introduced virtually every form of Theravāda and Mahāyāna to the United States. Mahāyāna devotees from Northeast Asia began arriving in the middle of the 19th century as part of the labor diaspora, a direct result of the end of the African slave trade. A hundred years later, their spiritual cohorts from Tibet, Mongolia, and Vietnam entered the United States as refugees and immigrants. Substantial numbers of Theravāda devotees arrived from Sri Lanka, Myanmar (Burma), Thailand, Laos, and Cambodia during the last quarter of the past century. The Hart-Celler Act of 1965, which did away with quotas based on national origin, eased the entry of Asian Buddhists into the United States.

The US Census Bureau, *Statistical Abstract of the United States: 2006,* estimates that there are 1,082,000 Buddhists in the United States. This figure is extrapolated from 50,281 random digit-dialed telephone surveys by the American Religious Identification Survey conducted in 2001. Somewhat earlier in 1994, Peter Jennings, on *ABC Nightly News*, estimated that American Buddhists number between 4 and 6 million individuals. Whatever the numbers, roughly 75%–80% are of Asian descent who inherited the

The US Census Bureau, Statistical Abstract of the United States: 2006, estimates that there are 1,082,000 Buddhists in the United States.

faith as a family tradition; the remaining 20%–25% are American converts, who should have no special difficulty negotiating the American health care system.

History

Siddhārtha Gautama (ca. 563-483 BCE), the founder of the Buddhist faith and community, was prince of a small kingdom that straddled the present-day border of Nepal and northeast India. By the second century BCE, Buddhism had a significant presence in most of India, Sri Lanka, and Central Asia. Buddhist culture entered China in the first century BCE, Korea by the middle of the fourth century, and Japan two centuries later. In the meantime, by the eighth century, Buddhist culture had extended its influence to continental and island Southeast Asia, where Theravāda eventually eclipsed Mahāyāna and is dominant today. Mahāyāna in the form of Vajrayāna, later called Tantric Buddhism, made its way to Tibet in the seventh century. Tibetan monks carried their faith to Mongolia in the 13th and again in the 16th centuries. Buddhism's success is attributed to its ability to acknowledge the validity of other indigenous spiritual traditions and its medical knowledge.

> *Buddhism's success is attributed to its ability to acknowledge the validity of other indigenous spiritual traditions and its medical knowledge.*

Beliefs and Doctrines

Siddhārtha Gautama began his spiritual journey with the question of human suffering that accompanies aging, sickness, and death. After 6 years of spiritual exercises, Gautama realized the Dharma, the truth of *pratītyasamutpāda*, dependent co-arising or interdependence, and became the Buddha—"the Enlightened One." The community that the Buddha founded remained a single unit for about 100 years after his passing when disagreements split the original community into the present-day Theravāda and Mahāyāna schools.

Theravāda and Mahāyāna differ in their respective understanding of *pratītyasamutpāda*, the ideological core of Buddhist thought and practice. *Pratītyasamutpāda* can be understood to be an extension of karma, the law of cause and effect. Both traditions link karma, or "action," with personal moral responsibility. An individual's present station in life is the result of the moral quality of karma that was generated in the past. Likewise, deeds committed in the present life affect an individual's future condition. Mahāyāna expanded this initial understanding of karma on the reality that, in an interdependent world, an individual does not live in a social or psychological vacuum. An individual's action is conditioned by multiple causes and conditions; further the karmic energy that one generates is mitigated by the interests and concerns of others and by the intrusion of other karmic forces that include historical and geopolitical forces that often thwart personal intent. Pure Land Buddhist teachings maintain that individuals who are helplessly caught up in powerful karmic flows can entrust themselves only to the great compassion of the Amida Buddha for spiritual liberation.

Pratītyasamutpāda is the ideological basis for compassion, a prime Buddhist virtue. The vision of an interdependent world means that all beings rise and fall as a single body; one should thus behave in ways that will benefit all others. Compassion is also established by enlightenment or wisdom. Enlightened knowing knows the suffering of others, which in turn quickens compassionate thoughts and acts.

> *Pratītyasamutpāda is the ideological basis for compassion, a prime Buddhist virtue. The vision of an interdependent world means that all beings rise and fall as a single body; one should thus behave in ways that will benefit all others.*

Death and Afterlife

The Buddha for his part refrained from answering questions concerning the afterlife or the origins of the universe; such speculations distract from the more immediate questions of human suffering—poverty, disease, and discrimination—that can be remedied through human effort. The popular imagination did not find much comfort in the Buddha's strict empiricism and skepticism of the "unproven" and "unknown" and very quickly transformed the idea of nirvana, the goal of the Buddhist project, into an ideal realm that is free of suffering. Although the historical Buddha is believed to have purged all worldly desires through spiritual discipline that spanned many rebirths and entered into nirvana at the time of his death, never to be reborn, in Theravāda cultures the ordinary devotee is content to achieve a better rebirth, usually associated with a higher socioeconomic status, by cultivating good works, avoiding evil, and purifying the mind. A favorable rebirth is facilitated by taking up the holy life in later stages of life, which prepares an individual to hold meritorious thoughts in the final critical moments before death.

Likewise, Japanese Pure Land Buddhism transformed the idea of nirvana into *Sukhāvatī*, or Pure Land, that is presided over by the Amida Buddha, whose great compassion welcomes all beings, even the most evil. Unlike the Theravāda devotee who must cultivate the mind over many lifetimes, any person who invokes the nembutsu with genuine sincerity, even the most wicked, will enter the Pure Land. The nembutsu is Amida Buddha's name in the form *Namu Amida Butsu*—I take refuge in the Buddha Amida.

Holidays and Observances

The Theravāda and Mahāyāna traditions observe different ritual calendars. The major Theravāda Buddhist observance is Vesakah Bucha (Tai), which marks the birth, enlightenment, and death of the Buddha; it is celebrated on the full moon of the second month of the lunar Hindu calendar, which corresponds to May in the Western calendar. Most Japanese Pure Land temples follow the Western calendar (some still follow the Chinese lunar calendar) and observe the birth of the Buddha on 8 April, his enlightenment on 8 December, and his death on 15 February. The other major Japanese Buddhist observance is Obon, which celebrates the homecoming of the deceased ancestors from the land of the spirits. Congregate worship is not an important feature in American Theravāda temples. During the past 100 years, Pure Land worship has evolved into a form that resembles a Protestant Christian service.

> *Most Japanese Pure Land temples follow the Western calendar (some still follow the Chinese lunar calendar) and observe the birth of the Buddha on 8 April, his enlightenment on 8 December, and his death on 15 February.*

Deathbed, Mortuary, and Memorial Rituals

Deathbed, mortuary, and memorial rituals in Thai-Lao Theravāda and Japanese Pure Land traditions have integrated non-Buddhist beliefs, most notably the belief in disembodied spirits or ghosts. This belief assumes that life and death is a continuum and that familial relationships and obligations continue between the living and the deceased.

When death is imminent in Theravāda cultures, clerics or lay elders may be invited to chant sections of the *Abhidhamma*, a ritual text, at the deathbed and offer words of encouragement to calm the mind of the dying. Exiting this life with a quiescent mind is essential for a favorable rebirth. Unexpected death due to a sudden illness, accident, or crime confuses the spirit of the deceased. Unprepared for death, the spirit clings to the corporal life and causes havoc by remaining nearby familiar haunts. Regardless of the circumstances of death, the living relatives will sponsor mortuary and regular memorial rituals to assist the deceased to understand his or her new life. Neglecting these obligations may result in illness, death, and other misfortunes on family members.

Unexpected death due to a sudden illness, accident, or crime confuses the spirit of the deceased. Unprepared for death, the spirit clings to the corporal life and causes havoc by remaining nearby familiar haunts.

Similarly, when death is imminent, a Pure Land cleric will reassure the individual of his or her birth in the Pure Land by chanting the *Amidakyō* (Smaller Sukhavati Sutra) and/or brief words of such promise. The chanting of the sutra is an opportunity for the dying to hear the teachings of the Buddha and to cultivate a genuine desire to be born in the Pure Land. Like in Theravāda cultures, the living descendants have a filial obligation to assist the deceased to transform himself or herself from a corporeal to a spiritual being (kami) by sponsoring mortuary and memorial observances. In return for such devotion, the ancestor protects and ensures the health and prosperity of the family. Failure to observe the memorial cycle and make offerings angers the deceased ancestors and is manifested in misfortune on their living descendents. The ritual cycle incorporates Indian Buddhist notions of karma and successive lives, Confucian ideas of filial piety and memorial tablets, and Shintō views of ancestorhood. Only the very devout continue to observe the memorial cycle in its entirety in the United States today; the ritual cycle has been abbreviated by the American experience.

Late-Life Celebrations

Both the Thai-Lao and Japanese observe late-life rituals that demonstrate intergeneration reciprocity and give elders milestones to look forward to. Thai-Lao cultures observe the *suebchata* or ceremony for the prolongation of life on the occasion of a person's sixtieth birthday and every twelfth year thereafter is marked for special celebration.[1] The family of a frail elder may also sponsor *sookwan*, a ritual to reenergize a person's spirit-essence by inviting all ancestors to assist in this task. These rituals may be performed by a cleric or an elder.

1. The 12-year cycle is adopted from the Chinese zodiac, which consists of 12 animals: rat, cow, tiger, rabbit, dragon, snake, horse, sheep, monkey, chicken, dog, and boar; and 5 elements: wood, fire, earth, metal, and water. Thus, every sixty-first year has the same animal and element symbol.

The late-life rituals and mortuary and memorial rites commonly observed by the Japanese and Japanese American community highlight the importance of filiality and the importance of family lineage. Birthdays at ages 60, 70, 77, 80, 88, 90, and 99 are especially significant milestones. The sixtieth birthday, *kanreki*, marks the completion of one life cycle according to the Chinese zodiac, and the beginning of a new cycle. The eighty-eighth year, *beijū*, is an especially auspicious occasion.

Gender Issues

Conceding that women possess the ability to ascend and realize the highest reaches of insight, the Buddha ordained women into the inner circle of his fledging community. The status of women in Buddhist communities has generally reflected prevailing sociopolitical attitudes of their respective host cultures. Theravāda nuns do not enjoy as much prestige as their male counterparts. Pure Land women clerics enjoy the same privileges as their male colleagues. In Theravāda cultures, monks are not to be touched by women.

Medical Theory

Buddhist medical theory understands mind and body to be a single unit. Illness of the body impacts mental health; similarly, mental illness directly affects physical well-being.

Buddhist medical theory understands mind and body to be a single unit. Illness of the body impacts mental health; similarly, mental illness directly affects physical well-being. Physical health is evidence of the balance among the four elements *(māhabhūta)*, usually earth (solid), water (wet), fire (hot), and wind (mobile), that constitute the corporal body. Illness arises when one or more of these elements undergoes radical change(s) that disturbs this fourfold equilibrium. Medical and pharmacologic therapies aim to maintain and restore physical and mental well-being that may be upset by diet, seasonal changes, and physical and emotional stresses. A wholesome lifestyle, proper diet, and meditation maintain balance of the four elements. Although disease is traced to empirical causes, the residual effects of karma (past action) is also a category of medical etiology. The residual effects of unwholesome past thoughts and deeds impact both present and future health and well-being.

Buddha traced much of physical illnesses and mental illness to poverty. Adequate nutrition, clothing, shelter, and health care optimize the possibility for education and spiritual development. The government has the responsibility to ensure wholesome living conditions by safeguarding the natural environment; by responsibly managing and distributing economic and other resources; by instituting effective public health policies; and by protecting the poor and dispossessed from exploitation. In keeping with the belief that prevention is the best guarantee against illness and disease, the Buddha urged moderation in all life activities, including spiritual exercises.

Buddha traced much of physical illnesses and mental illness to poverty.

Advance Directives

Buddhist medicine has no special position on do-not-resuscitate orders or on nutrition and hydration at the end of life. Medical decisions are guided by compassion and kindness for the well-being of the dying that will ensure a peaceful death. Although the Buddhist teaching of *ahimsa,* or no-harming, did much to encourage vegetarianism, except for the most devout, most Buddhists are omnivorous.

Medical decisions are guided by compassion and kindness for the well-being of the dying that will ensure a peaceful death.

Reflecting the belief that the Buddha began his spiritual quest with the question of human suffering that accompanies aging, sickness, and death, Buddhist clerics promote the appreciation of the fragility of the human condition. Still, the medical professional should be cautious about informing a patient of a terminal prognosis, because many Japanese believe that he or she will lose the will to live. Theravāda devotees are generally more open to such a prognosis because of their belief in karma.

Buddhist clerics promote the appreciation of the fragility of the human condition.

Buddhist Literature

The sacred canon, or the *Tripitika,* comprises the sutras (the direct teachings of the Buddha), the sastras (the learned commentaries), and the *Vinaya* (the monastic codes). The Theravāda cannon is preserved in Pali, a language related to Sanskrit. The Mahāyāna *Tripitaka* exists primarily in translations of Chinese, Tibetan, and other Central Asian languages. It has been estimated that only about 7% of Buddhist literature has been rendered into English.

Titles of Spiritual Functionaries

The Theravāda cleric is called *ahjan*, teacher, or *luang-po*, venerable father, in Lao-Tai. The official title for the Jodōshinshu cleric is *kaikyōshi*,
Dharma-master, but devotees normally refer to their spiritual leader as
sensei, teacher, a more affectionate title.

CASE STUDY **1**	**The Power of Faith**

Objectives

1. Consider the efficacy of faith and meditation in controlling pain and easing depression and family tension.
2. Understand the therapeutic role that the *nembutsu*, invoking the name of the Amida Buddha, might have.

Mr. M., a *nisei kibei* (a person born in the United States but raised in Japan), suffered from persistent chronic pain for the last 20 years of his life. In an attempt to relieve the pain, during a 9 ½-hour operation, surgeons at the Mayo Clinic successfully removed a tumor that had wrapped itself around his lower spinal cord. The procedure saved his life, but pain remained. Mr. M. lost the ability to walk and was confined to a wheelchair. His physicians advised that the pain would be mitigated over time and did not prescribe addictive opiates. Passing away at 73 years, Mr. M. outlived his prognosis by 10 years.

Mr. M.'s pain caused him to verbally abuse Mrs. M., his primary caregiver, who contemplated a divorce. She was at her wits' end, until a visiting Jodōshin cleric brought a copy of the *Teaching of the Buddha* and suggested that she read it as a way of relieving her frustration. Reading the book, she had many questions, which she would then ask her husband, a devout Pure Land devotee, for clarification. Mrs. M. noticed he would become noticeably calmer while explaining the passages and would be able to sleep throughout the night. Mrs. M. recalls asking "What is the meaning of karma?" and "Please explain the Noble Truth of Suffering." She would read and reread the *Teaching of the Buddha*, not for her own edification but for questions to ask. When her husband slept, she too could rest. Mr. M. was greatly distressed that he was unable to utter the *nembutsu*. "But at night I hear you reciting the *nembutsu* while you are asleep." Mrs. M. noticed that chanting sutra passages also helped to ease his pain.

Mr. and Mrs. M., like most Japanese Americans in the continental United States, were uprooted and sent to relocation centers for the duration of World War II. As a result, the Japanese community harbors great distrust of governmental authority. How much of this distrust is transferred to the medical profession? Mr. and Mrs. M. chanced on their palliative therapy when a visiting cleric passed on The Teaching of the Buddha. Would spiritual therapies be effective for a less devout person? What role does chanting and meditation have in medical therapy?

Mr. and Mrs. M. are bilingual and bicultural. Having been born and lived most of their lives in the United States, they are more adept in negotiating the American health care system.

Question:
1. What are some of the layers of spiritual culture that may have helped the family in dealing with the American medical system?

CASE STUDY **2**	**Porously Laminated Spiritual Layers**

Objectives
1. Consider multiple spiritual layers that guide the patient's attempt to control her pain.
2. Consider the appropriateness of the concurrent use of alternative therapies.

Mrs. C., a 43-year-old Laotian-Thai, is receiving concurrent chemotherapy and radiation therapy for cancer of the lower left lung from an American-trained Thai physician. She was a heavy smoker. Fearful of the spreading conflict in Vietnam, she fled with her family from a remote mountain village in 1975 for Thailand; she was 11 at the time. The family settled temporarily at the Sabtun Refugee Camp. After being granted refugee status, the family relocated to California in 1980. Like most immigrants, Mrs. C. relies on modern American medicine, traditional herbal therapies, and *samatha-vipaśyanā*, a Theravāda meditation technique that she learned from her father, a traditional healer. She can communicate in English but does not have sufficient command of the language to fully express her feelings.

Theravāda Buddhism is the nominal faith she grew up with. The nearest temple was a day away on foot. She also observed the animist rituals honoring the spirits of trees and rocks, and she is aware of and communicates with the *phii*, spirits that co-inhabit her world. She recently reminded the disembodied spirit of her father that he is no longer of this world and that he should not interfere with her life. She became a Roman Catholic while residing in a refugee camp. When asked why she converted, she responded: "We siblings did what my mother told us to do; we did not understand." After moving to her present home, she joined the Assembly of God Church. Although she believes in a Christian God, who is "bigger than all things," she wonders about her karmic past for her present condition. She is grateful for her family's support and continues to fight her cancer so she can take care of her family.

Mrs. C. studied English for 3 years after relocating to the United States. She left school to work. She is happy that her radiation oncologist can explain the rationale and progress of her treatment in her native tongue. "He understands me," she said with delight. Under the best of circumstances, cross-cultural communication is difficult; how much more when one is ill and trying to negotiate an unfamiliar medical system? What can be done to bridge language and cultural divides? It takes years of training to become competent in a second language, even longer to master medical terminology and the underlying concepts.

Mrs. C. freely discusses her alternative therapies with her Thai radiation-oncologist but has never mentioned their use to her primary care physician for fear of being told to abandon them.

Buddhism regards a day-old child and a centenarian to be of the same age. No matter how old or young we may be, today may be our last. Life is indeed transient and very uncertain. How may such a belief in the fragileness of life impact daily decisions and medical treatment?

Questions:

1. How does the American medical system deal with complementary therapies? Is it possible to integrate alternative therapies and meditation?
2. What procedures are in place to consult with traditional healers and spiritual advisers?

Ronald Y. Nakasone, PhD
Vitune Vongtama, MD

References

Aung MH. *Folk Elements in Burmese Buddhism.* Rangoon, Myanmar: U Hla Maung Buddha Sasana Press; 1959.

Buddhism in America. Available at: http://en.wikipedia.org/wiki (accessed December 2006).

Buddhist views on biotechnology. In: Murray TH, Mehlman, MJ (eds). *Encyclopedia of Ethical, Legal & Policy Issues in Biotechnology.* New York: Wiley; 2000.

Chappell DW, Tsomo KK (eds). *Living and Dying in Buddhist Cultures.* Honolulu: Buddhist Studies Program, University of Hawaii.

Charles K Hasegawa, Minister, Buddhist Church of Stockton, CA; Interview, April 2007.

Coward H, Ratanakul P (eds). *A Cross-cultural Dialogue on Health Care Ethics.* Waterloo, Canada: Wilfrid Laurier University Press; 1999.

Demiéville P. *Buddhism and Healing.* Lanham, MD: University of America Press (trans. Mark Tatz); 1985.

Heng Sure, Abbot, Berkeley Buddhist Monastary, Berkeley, CA; Interview, April 2007.

Hughes JJ, Keown D. Buddhism and medical ethics: a bibliographic introduction. *J Buddhist Ethics* vol. 2. Available at: http://www.changesurfer.com/Bud/BudBio-Eth.html.

Ishii Y. *Sangha, State, and Society: Thai Buddhism in History*. Honolulu: University of Hawaii Press; 1986.

Kakar S. *Shamans, Mystics and Doctors, a Psychological Inquiry into India and its Healing Traditions*. Delhi: Oxford University Press; 1982.

Nakasone RY. Buddhist issues in end-of-life decision making. In: Braun K, et al (eds). *Issues in End-of-Life Decision Making*. New York: Sage Publications; 1999.

Namihira E. Japanese concepts and attitude toward human remains. In: Hoshino K (ed). *Japanese and Western Bioethics, Studies in Moral Diversity*. Dordrecht, The Netherlands: Kluwer Academic Publishers; 1997.

Pali Text Society. *Casket of Medicine*. The Oxford: The Pali Text Society; 2002 (trans. Jinadasa Liyanaratne).

Phra Maha Prasert, Abbot, Wat Buddhanusorn, Fremont, CA; Interview, April 2007.

Prebish C, Tanaka KK, (eds). *The Faces of Buddhism in America*. Berkeley: University of California Press; 1998:1.

Ratanakul P. Bioethics in Thailand: The struggle for Buddhist solutions. *J Med Philos* 1988;13:301–312.

Tambiah SJ. Buddhism and the Spirit Cults in North-East Thailand. Cambridge: Cambridge University Press; 1970.

Terwiel, BJ. *Monks and Magic, an Analysis of Religious Ceremonies in Central Thailand*. Bangkok, Thailand: White Lotus; 1994.

Umehara T. The Japanese view of the hereafter. *Japan Echo* 1989;16(3).

US Census Bureau, *Statistical Abstract of the United States: 2006*. Self-described religious identification of adult population: 1990 and 2001, Table 69. Available at: http://www.census.gov/compendia/statab/population/pop.pdf (accessed December 2006).

Zysk KG. *Asceticism and Healing in Ancient India, Medicine in the Buddhist Monastery*. Delhi, India: Oxford University Press; 1991.

CHAPTER 4

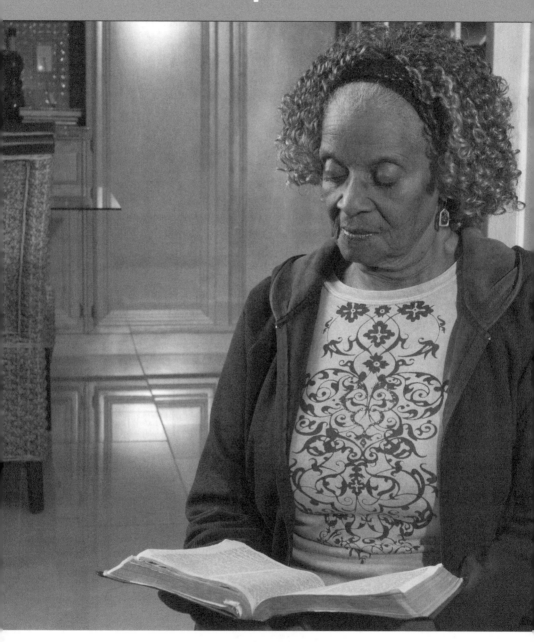

Christianity

When people in the United States are asked what religious group they are most likely to identify with, approximately 80% say they are Christian. However, Christianity comprises diverse sects, and what each individual Christian might need during a time of emotional or physical crisis is too often overlooked.

Dimitri Papovich is a 92-year-old man presenting in a faith-based community hospital with a hip fracture on January 3. During his initial assessment on the unit he noted a staff member taking down the Christmas decorations and began to protest. He kept saying, "How can you take down Christmas when it has not happened yet?" While this seemed to be the only indication of disorientation, because of his persistence, he was presumed to be confused and disoriented, and was labeled so by the staff. His English was somewhat deficient, which made his protests more difficult to understand. As staff began to disregard his complaints, he began to escalate his concerns to the point that the nursing staff called for and were given an order for sedation and physical restraints. The next morning when he was being prepared for surgery, Mr. Papovich's daughter arrived carrying a Christmas tree and decorations for his room. She quietly explained to the staff that Mr. Papovich is an Eastern Orthodox Christian. In this tradition, the Eastern calendar is used to determine the date for Christmas, and this year it was in early January.

No one in this faith-based Protestant hospital unit in this major metropolitan city had any idea that some Christian groups celebrate Christmas on a different date; therefore, this elderly gentleman was assumed to have dementia, because, after all, he was old.

History

Christianity was founded by Jesus Christ. He was born about 4 BCE and died about 30 CE.[1] In a short span of time, his disciples went from being Jewish Christians to Christian Jews and then to a separate group of Christians. This transition occurred between 30 and 70 CE. Within 50 years of the death of Christ, a new community had been formed with its own beliefs and leadership. The new leadership and the belief system are clearly documented in the New Testament.

> *Within 50 years of the death of Christ, a new community had been formed with its own beliefs and leadership.*

Christianity stands on the shoulders of the Jewish tradition, which in many ways is its older brother and sister. Many of the prayers and worship services have their roots in the Jewish faith. Christianity accepts the covenant that was given to Abraham and Sarah as valid and enduring. What Christianity adds to the original covenant is the new and eternal covenant with Jesus Christ.

Jesus is believed to be the Son of God. Through his Incarnation, he becomes man. In many ways, this is a radical change for Judaism. As a monotheistic religion (along with Christianity and Islam), the belief in one God is challenged if Jesus is also God. Christians believe that God is one (monotheism), yet God is also Trinity (Father, Son, and Holy Spirit).

There are four key mysteries in Christianity: the Incarnation (God becomes man in Jesus Christ); the Trinity; the resurrection of Jesus from the dead on Easter Sunday; and the Body of Christ (the physical body, the resurrected body, and the community of believers). These mysteries are fundamental to understanding how Christianity is different than Judaism and why a new community was established.

The Christian community grew and developed in the Roman Empire. In many ways, the community benefited from the Empire and the good modes of communication it afforded. The community also ran afoul of the Empire when Christians refused to offer worship to the Roman gods and goddesses. With the conquest of Constantine in 314 CE, Christianity became the state religion.

> *With the conquest of Constantine in 314 CE, Christianity became the state religion.*

---

1. Most of the major religions in the world have developed calendars, most of which are much older than the Christian Calendar. However, the Christian Calendar has been adopted for general use today. Since it is employed by many faith traditions, instead of BC (Before Christ) and AD (After Christ), it is appropriate to substitute BCE (Before the Common Era) and CE (the Common Era).

Christianity remained a unified body until 1054 CE when two Christian groups emerged. One group was loyal to Rome, and the other was focused in Constantinople (Istanbul). The split occurred for both theological and political reasons. The major theological issue is that of the *Filioque*, which is a technical issue concerning the procession of the Holy Spirit. The political issues involved the question of the authority of the Pope, the use of leavened bread in the Mass, and the question of married clergy. From a geographical perspective, the dividing line often went through the Balkans and up into Russia. Those who allied with Rome become known as Roman Catholics, and those who allied with Constantinople become known as Eastern Rite Catholics.

Controversies and minor divisions have been a part of the Christian traditions since the early church. However, the next major split took place in 1517 CE, when Martin Luther nailed his 95 theses to the door of the Wittenberg Chapel. John Calvin and Ulrich Zwingli began their reformation efforts 30 years later; with a succession of others, including John Wesley in England, this constituted the period known as the Protestant reformation.

> *Controversies and minor divisions have been a part of the Christian traditions since the early church.*

Once again both theological and political issues were involved. The major theological issue involved the question of how one was saved. Is it purely a gift from God, or does the individual have to cooperate in some fashion? Political issues revolved around the authority of the Pope, the appointment of local leadership, and the use of the vernacular in the worship services. If communications had been better at the time, probably much of this could have been avoided. Other efforts at restoration have taken place since, some particularly affecting Christianity in the United States.

This division had a major impact on Europe. It led to the Wars of Religion in the 1600s and would eventually be played out in the territories that were explored and claimed as colonies by the European governments.

Denominations

Approximately 30,000 different groups or denominations of people around the world call themselves Christian. According to a University of New York study, 79.8% of people in the United States consider

According to a University of New York study, 79.8% of people in the United States consider themselves to be Christian.

themselves to be Christian. According to one source, there are over 214 Protestant denominations in the United States alone. In this context, it can be helpful to find groups of denominations. Various Christian denominations and sects can be grouped in a variety of ways. One approach identifies six groups: Catholic, Episcopal, Presbyterian, Congregational, Pentecostals, and Restorationists.[2]

Catholic

The Catholic group includes the Roman Catholic denomination, along with the Orthodox traditions; Eastern Orthodox, Russian Orthodox, and Greek Orthodox denominations are the larger groups in the United States. Roman Catholicism is the largest single group of Christians both in the world and in the United States. Although estimates of the sizes of the various denominations vary, Roman Catholics are estimated to constitute 25.9% of all Christians in the United States. In the United States, Orthodox Christians constitute 0.3% of the population. In the Catholic traditions, a central authority, or Pope, is *the* authority, particularly for ecclesial decision making. Churches vary in their structure and beliefs, but each recognizes this hierarchal authority and is structured to carry this authority to the entire world.

Churches vary in their structure and beliefs, but each recognizes this hierarchal authority and is structured to carry this authority to the entire world.

Episcopal

The Episcopal denominations include the Episcopal, Lutheran, and Methodist denominations. Methodists constitute approximately 7.2%, Lutherans 4.9%, and Episcopalian or Anglican Christians approximately 1.8% of Christians in the United States. Within the Episcopal denominations, authority resides in councils of heads of regions known as bishops.

Presbyterian

Presbyterian polity, which is best represented by the various Presbyterian and Reformed Church denominations in the United States,

---

2. Our approach to categorizing Protestant denominations is based on: Robinson BA. 2003. Christian Meta-Groups: One Method of Sorting the Thousands of Christian Denominations into Groups. In: Ontario Consultants on Religious Tolerance. www.religioustolerance.org/chr_pent.htm (accessed April 21, 2007) with modifications by James W. Ellor.

reflects 2.8% of Christians. These denominations are connected, in that there is one set of standards that is to be followed by all churches. However, following the insights of John Calvin, instead of leadership coming from individuals, such as a bishop, this polity is run by committees, organized in local and regional groups.

Congregational

Congregational polity is reflective of organizations in which ultimate authority is in each local church or congregation. While many have associations such as the various Baptist Associations, each church retains significant independence for governance. The largest example of this group is the Baptists, who constitute 17.2% of Christians in the United States.

> *Congregational polity is reflective of organizations in which ultimate authority is in each local church or congregation.*

Pentecostal

The holiness movement, the roots of which are in the Methodist tradition, spawned the various Pentecostal denominations. Today, there are over 177 Pentecostal or Charismatic denominations constituting approximately 2.2% of Christians in the United States. A defining feature of this group is the emphasis on the gifts of the spirit. One such is the belief in prayer in tongues. Although often misunderstood by people from other Christian faith groups, this practice is supported by Christian Scripture and is not reflective of any sort of mental illness.

> *The holiness movement, the roots of which are in the Methodist tradition, spawned the various Pentecostal denominations.*

Restorationist

Finally, the Restorationist faith traditions emerged in the 1800s and 1900s. Much like the original reformation traditions, this group seeks the "true" God, who they feel has been abandoned by other Christians. This group includes the Jehovah's Witnesses, 0.7%; Seventh-day Adventists, 0.4%; and the Church of the Latter-Day Saints or Mormon denomination, 1.4% of Christians in the United States. Each of these denominations reflects unique beliefs that need to be understood in terms of their impact on health care.

Four variables cut across the six categories of congregations. The first is that of Pentecostal gifts of the spirit. While there is a Pentecostal group of denominations, there are also clusters of people who identify with the Pentecostal or gifts of the spirit movement within many of

TABLE 1 Conceptual Matrix for Denominational Analysis

	Pentecostal	Mystical	Culture	Race	Out of Date
Catholic					
Episcopal					
Presbyterian					
Congregational					
Pentecostal					
Restorationist					

the traditional Roman Catholic, Episcopal, and Presbyterian traditions. The second are those who view the church through the mystics. Found more often in the Catholic and Episcopal groups, the mystical traditions focus on the mystical relationship and power of God. The third group reflects the culture of origin of the congregation. People emigrating from other countries to the United States frequently brought their culture with them as a part of their faith. Thus, many Lutheran congregations identify with various German and Scandinavian countries, and some Catholics identify with various Eastern European countries.

Race is also a variable. Some Protestant denominations, such as the African Methodist Episcopal denomination, sprung up at the time of the Civil War as faith communities for former slaves. Other churches, for example those in the Baptist denomination, simply developed individual churches within the larger denominational family of churches. Finally, an analysis of older adults and their involvement in a church reflects that they cling to the traditions of the church that was a part of their childhood. For example, in the Roman Catholic Church during the 1960s, important changes were made, particularly in the prayers offered at a time of illness. Before the meeting of the Second Vatican Council, these prayers were referred to as "last rites" (ie, prayers for a person as she or he was dying). Today, these prayers are understood as pastoral care for the sick and dying and are sometimes referred to as "prayers for the sick." Older adults may still request "last rites" and be disturbed that they are not treated in the "old way."

Some Protestant denominations, such as the African Methodist Episcopal denomination, sprung up at the time of the Civil War as faith communities for former slaves.

Older adults may still request "last rites" and be disturbed that they are not treated in the "old way."

The role of women in ministry may be difficult for some older adults in Protestant churches to accept. Older adults may also have difficulty adjusting to other changes in the various denominations that have involved prayers, hymns, and liturgies. At times of illness, seniors may revert back to these traditions or request the older versions of them.

Important Holidays

The most important holy day for Christians is Easter Sunday. This is the day that Christ rose from the dead. The second most important day is December 25, which is the birth of Christ (his Incarnation). These two days are celebrated by five of the six groups of denominations. The exception is the Jehovah's Witnesses in the Restorationist group, who strictly follow the Bible; because Jesus never celebrated his birthday in scripture, they do not do so. There are two important seasons for Christians. These are Advent, a 4-week period before Christmas, and Lent, a 40-day period before Easter. These seasons are marked by extra prayer, fasting, and alms giving.

Particularly for Catholic and Episcopal groups, other important dates are the feast of the Epiphany (January 6), the feast of All Souls (October 31), and All Saints Day (November 1). In the Latino culture, All Souls is celebrated as the Day of the Dead (Dios de los Muertos).

Sacred Objects and Scriptures

In Christianity, the sacred scripture is the Bible. Christians accept both the Old and New Testament. The books of the Bible are God's self-communication with humanity. Christians believe that the books are inspired—that is, that they are written under the guidance of the Holy Spirit. The words of the Bible were not dictated; rather, the thoughts were inspired by God, and then the individual writer used all of his insight to write the text. Although errors concerning cosmology and historical sequencing may exist, there are no errors concerning moral truth. Some groups of Christians interpret the text as being literally true; most however, understand the text to contain moral truth and guidance. Some variance also

In Christianity, the sacred scripture is the Bible. Christians accept both the Old and New Testament. The books of the Bible are God's self-communication with humanity.

Some groups of Christians interpret the text as being literally true; most however, understand the text to contain moral truth and guidance.

exists in which books are included in the Bible. Several books of the Old Testament, known as the Apocrypha, are included by Catholic groups but often not by Presbyterian and Congregational groups.

The most important sacred object is the cross, which is the symbol of Christ's victory over death. A cross is present in most Christian homes and places of worship. This symbol is important across Christian traditions, although it is presented differently by various groups.

Catholic Christians have a number of sacred symbols. These include holy water (blessed water that reminds the individual of Baptism and the washing away of sin); icons (pictures of Christ, Mary, and the saints); the rosary (a series of beads with a cross), used to recall the mysteries of faith; the Sacred Host (a wafer) that Catholics believe becomes the body and blood of Christ when it is consecrated at Mass; holy cards and statues of Christ, Mary, and the saints; and prayer books.

Protestant groups are divided regarding baptism. For Presbyterian and Episcopal groups, baptism is performed by sprinkling the water on the person to be baptized. In some Congregational and many Pentecostal groups, baptism is performed only on people who are of an age to make a personal decision about their own baptism and consists of immersion in a pool of water.

Clergy

For the Roman Catholic community, the principal leader is the pope. He appoints local leaders (bishops), who ordain priests and deacons. The tradition is very hierarchical. Members of the laity are not ordained. In the Eastern Rite tradition, the principal leader is the patriarch. There are a number of patriarchs, and they share leadership in a collegial way. Patriarchs appoint bishops, who in turn ordain priests. There is, however, no one spokesman.

In the Catholic tradition, an important leadership role is played by professed religious women (sisters). They have a very important role in providing care for ill and aging populations.

Three types of authority can be used by Christian clergy: administrative, spiritual, and ritual. Parishioners view their pastor as the person who is paid to run the church. Many pastors in smaller churches are part-time; however, the critical variable for the health care provider is the perception of the parishioner. Is the pastor perceived to be in charge of the church? The second variable is that of spiritual leader.

Carl Menninger noted that there are two types of therapists who are perceived to have Magic to offer their clients: the psychiatrist with his or her pills, and the minister with his or her relationship with God. At times of crisis, clergy are often the first people contacted for help; parishioners are often seeking the comfort that comes with their perception of the pastor's relationship with God (however God is perceived). Finally, clergy are the keepers of the rituals of the church. This includes authority to offer rituals that signify entrance into the church and forgiveness and can help interpret the word of God. Older adults endow their clergy with symbols of power. It is critical for health care providers to understand these perceptions, because in many cases these beliefs are also supported by the structure and beliefs of their church.

At times of crisis, clergy are often the first people contacted for help.

Religious Basis for Views of Health and Disease

All Christians see the body as good and sacred. In the creation story (Genesis 1-2), man and woman are created not only good but very good. They are created in the image and likeness of God. Therefore, there is a great deal of respect for the body, and there is an obligation to care for the body.

In an earlier time, some Christians viewed illness as punishment; however, this is strongly refuted by Christ. In the ninth chapter of Saint John's gospel, there is the story of a man born blind. The disciples ask if he is blind because of a personal failure or because his parents were sinners. Jesus responds that the blindness is not the result of failure on anyone's part. Rather, the sickness or limitation is an opportunity for God to demonstrate his healing power and an opportunity for us to provide care for those in need.

Health is a gift from God so that we can accomplish the work that God has given us. We become stewards of the body and have an obligation to treat the body with care. We should avoid those things that would put the body at undue risk.

Sickness is a natural part of life. At some point, the physical body will begin to decline, and sickness will eventually lead to death. While it is expected that Christians will make an attempt to

While it is expected that Christians will make an attempt to fight the sickness, a time will come when further interventions are burdensome and the prognosis for restored health is not present.

fight the sickness, a time will come when further interventions are burdensome and the prognosis for restored health is not present. At that point, Christians are permitted and encouraged to let life and death take their natural course.

One group within the Restorationist denominations stands out in their view of illness and medicine. The Jehovah's Witnesses do not believe in blood transfusions. Based on the Biblical precedents of the Old Testament, Jehovah's Witnesses believe that infusing another person's blood defiles the body.

Dietary Restrictions

Christians believe that all food is part of God's creation and, therefore, is good.

There are few if any dietary restrictions. Christians believe that all food is part of God's creation and, therefore, is good.

Catholics who are in good health and younger than 60 years old are asked to reduce their food intake on Ash Wednesday (the beginning of the Lenten season) and on Good Friday (the day Christ died). Catholics are also required to refrain from eating meat on the Fridays during Lent. Eastern Rite Catholics have a more restrictive fast than Roman Catholics. All of these may be waived if the health of the patient requires a different diet.

Few Presbyterian, Congregational, or Pentecostal groups have any dietary restrictions. However, individual ethnic groups sometimes observe those also important to Catholics.

Gender Considerations

Christians believe that men and women are created in God's image and that they are created equally. Both have the same rights and privileges, and neither is to be discriminated against or taken advantage of. All are children of God.

Women play a critical ministerial role in education, health care services, and pastoral care for the aged, sick, and dying.

Catholic worship services have gender-specific roles, with only men being ordained as priests or deacons. Only priests can celebrate the Mass, hear confessions, and anoint the sick. Women play a critical ministerial role in education, health care services, and pastoral care for the aged, sick, and dying. Women often serve as ministers of the Eucharist and bring the sacred host to the hospital and other health care centers.

In many Protestant traditions, women may be ordained and are permitted to conduct the worship services. Episcopal and Presbyterian groups generally do ordain women. However, there is greater variance among the Congregational and Pentecostal groups. The United Church of Christ ordains women, but only some groups of Baptists do so. Health care practitioners should understand that regardless of whether the pastor is a woman or a man, the key to understanding her or his role reflects the three roles outlined above. Does the patient understand his or her pastor to have administrative, spiritual, and/or ritual authority?

Beliefs about Death and Dying

Christians believe that they were created for eternal life with God. The earthly existence is a prelude to eternal existence. There is a natural cycle of birth, growth and development, decline, and death. The Christian life does not end with death; rather, there is the belief in a resurrection from the dead and an eternal life with God.

Although no one should suffer for the sake of suffering and while all that is reasonable should be done to alleviate suffering, Christians know that suffering is part of life. It is through the suffering and death of Jesus Christ that humanity has been restored to friendship with God.

Suffering is an opportunity to be conformed more completely to Christ. If Christians pattern their lives on his, they believe that they will also be raised to life with him. In a pastoral letter written by John Paul II, entitled *Salvifici Dolores*, the Pope wrote eloquently about the redemptive meaning of suffering.

Suffering is an opportunity to be conformed more completely to Christ.

Death is not punishment; rather, it provides the doorway for transition from the earthly and limited existence to an eternal existence. Christians believe that they are created both body and soul. The body is limited to an earthly existence, but the soul will endure forever. Christians believe they will be raised both body and soul but that the new body will be a spiritualized body.

On death, Christians experience a judgment. Those who chose to do God's will will be raised to heaven and eternal life; those who did God's will imperfectly will experience a time in purgatory (a place in which separation from God is temporary); and those who refused to respond to God's invitation will experience hell. Hell is an eternal separation from God.

Heaven for the Christian is not so much a place as it is eternal life with God.

Heaven for the Christian is not so much a place as it is eternal life with God. The resurrected Christian will be with God and share in God's love eternally. Because God always lives in the present, eternity is not a long period of time. Rather, it is an opportunity to live in the eternal presence of God. Time takes on a new dimension, and we move from chronological time to *kairos*. This is a time that knows no limits and that affords the individual an unlimited opportunity to behold God.

Catholic Christians believe that there should be prayers for the dead. They offer Mass for the happy repose of the dead and believe that through their prayers and sacrifices, they can alleviate some of the time of separation for the souls in purgatory. Because all are members of the Body of Christ, they believe that they can still assist other members of the Body. This is often referred to as the communion of saints.

In contrast, Presbyterian and Congregational Christians understand that one goes to heaven only by the grace of God. Once death has occurred, nothing further can influence this decision, so prayers are for family members and their adjustment to the loss of the loved one.

Healing Ceremonies and Rituals

In the Catholic community, the healing ritual that the health care professional is most likely to encounter is the Rite of Anointing. Older patients and their families may refer to this as the "Last Rites." This ritual is practiced by many across the Protestant communities but with less consistency. It depends on the individual clergyperson and/or parishioner as to whether it is adopted.

The Church provides a series of rituals for those who are sick as well as for those who are dying, which is referred to as pastoral care of the sick.

Before the Church reforms that were instituted in the mid- and late- 1960s, a dying patient would receive this anointing just before death. Indeed, when the priest arrived it was often a signal to the patient that death was imminent. This anointing is now seen as part of a larger responsibility toward the sick.

The Church provides a series of rituals for those who are sick as well as for those who are dying, which is referred to as pastoral care of the sick. The Church provides this special care from the time that an illness becomes serious (ie, any illness that could lead to death). Old age is itself seen as an opportunity for anointing. Prayers are provided for children, those facing surgery, and for the dying. This care is referred to in the Letter of James (5:14–15) and in Mark (6:13). A careful reading of these texts indicates that prayer and anointing were already part of the Jewish tradition. The Christian community has updated and carried this ritual forward.

The person is anointed on the forehead as well as on the palms of the hands. This anointing is to remind the person of the anointing that was received in Baptism and of Christ's anointing. From a theological perspective, the Catholic Church teaches that the individual is restored to one's baptismal innocence. The person is thus in the best possible condition to encounter God. The rite always provides spiritual healing, and, if it is God's will, it may also provide physical healing. Because the person may receive this anointing more than once, everything should be done to ensure that this is provided before significant surgery and certainly before death. If death is imminent, the person should have the opportunity to celebrate the Sacrament of Penance and to receive the Eucharist.

The rite always provides spiritual healing, and, if it is God's will, it may also provide physical healing.

Most Presbyterian and Congregational denominations encourage prayer and the reading of scripture at times when healing is needed. The laying on of hands is one common ritual in which friends come together with the person who is sick and simply form a circle around the patient and pray together for God to heal the individual.

Views on Do-Not-Resuscitate

It is hoped that all older adults will have spoken with their spouse and children about their desire with respect to resuscitation. In living wills and in durable power of attorney, older adults can have established the conditions under which they would accept such care. The Christian community teaches that such care should be used when it is reasonable and when it will not impose an undue burden.

In an earlier era, Catholic Christians used the words "ordinary" and "extraordinary" care. However, when dealing with a worldwide community and the rapid advances in health care, these words often can mean very different things. In 1980, the Catholic Church issued a declaration on euthanasia (*Jura et bona*). In this pioneering work, the Church developed the concepts of benefit and burden. Thus, the patient should receive and accept all care that is beneficial and that does not impose an undue burden. However, the person is free to refuse any care that is burdensome and "just prolonging life." The person may be removed from any artificial means of support when it is deemed to be unduly burdensome. In other words, it is not necessary or desirable that every possible effort be used to prolong life, and one is not required to use every possible protocol to extend life.

> *The patient should receive and accept all care that is beneficial and that does not impose an undue burden.*

Some debate exists in the Catholic community regarding nutrition and hydration. One group sees it as ordinary care, permitting the withdrawal of nutrition and hydration if death is imminent, or if the person is no longer able to assimilate the nutrition. A much larger group, and one that refers to papal teaching, views nutrition and hydration as medical treatment that the patient or family is free to refuse. They see the spiritual purpose of life as more important than a mere temporal extension of life. In every case, the patient should receive palliative care and, to the extent possible, pain and suffering should be alleviated. Thus, it is not necessary or desirable to keep the patient alive under any circumstances. However, at no time may the person or the health care provider intentionally terminate life. Because life is sacred and because we are stewards and not owners of the body, only a natural death is permitted.

> *Because life is sacred and because we are stewards and not owners of the body, only a natural death is permitted.*

Presbyterian and Congregational groups of Christians are less consistent in these matters. Do-not-resuscitate orders are often more personal for the patient and his or her family.

Care After Death

Once death has occurred, prayers are offered for the deceased and/or for the family. The body should then be prepared for burial. In most cases, a wake service is held, often for 2 to 3 days. It is an opportunity for family and friends to mourn and to support each other.

For Catholic Christians, a Mass of the Resurrection is celebrated. If for some reason a Mass cannot be celebrated before interment, a memorial Mass can be celebrated at a later date. For the Catholic Christian, the body should be interred. In recent years, the Catholic Church has permitted cremation; however, the cremated body should be interred.

It is important for the Christian community to support the family after the death of a loved one. This is done through a "ministry of presence," as well as through holding the deceased and the family in prayer.

For Protestant Christians, it is more common for the wake to take place immediately before the funeral. The person and her or his family may also decide not to have a wake. In some instances, a memorial service takes place after the burial rather than a funeral service.

| CASE STUDY **1** | **Multiple Faiths, Multiple Views** |

Objectives
1. Examine the health care practices of different religious traditions and how they can be in conflict with both medicine and each other.
2. Better understand the role of a belief in an afterlife in making health care decisions.

In his book *How We Die,* Sherwin Nuland notes that no one dies of old age. In our sophisticated society, we have the ability to categorize every death. We can maintain statistical charts and document every intervention. In many ways, we are uncomfortable in saying that the body just "wore out." When we say there is no intervention, it seems as if we failed because we did not try some additional protocol.

Mrs. Thomas is 78 years old, and she lives in the assisted-living portion of a Continuum of Care Retirement Community. Her husband of 15 years has Alzheimer's disease and lives in the dementia unit at the same facility. This is a second marriage for both Mrs. Thomas and her husband. Her first husband died 20 years ago of a sudden heart attack. His first wife died 16 years ago of breast cancer. Will Thomas had done everything possible for his first wife. The minute her cancer was discovered, he flew into action, hiring the best surgeons with the most advanced techniques; she lived for 3 years after diagnosis. He never regretted his efforts to save her after nearly 40 years of marriage. When his second wife was diagnosed with cancer 7 years ago, he had done the same thing. He hired the best surgeons, and she had received state-of-the art care.

Recently, Mrs. Thomas was diagnosed with metastatic cancer of the liver. She was told that she had approximately 6 months to live if she did nothing, but not a lot longer even if she did because the cancer had spread.

Mrs. Thomas had been baptized in a Baptist Church when she was 12 years old. She remembers her own enthusiasm for attending Sunday school and the fellowship she had with her friends. However, she married a man who was not connected to his Congregational church, and the two of them fell away from any faith tradition until they were in their mid thirties when they joined the Jehovah's Witness congregation. They were practicing Jehovah's Witnesses until her husband died. When she married Mr. Thomas, she joined the Presbyterian Church. She was deeply conflicted during her first bout with cancer because the surgery required a blood transfusion, but she went along with it in obedience to her second husband.

Throughout her faith journey, Mrs. Thomas clung to the promises made by her Baptist pastor that she would some day have eternal life. She seemed to feel that it did not matter what church she attended— that promise was hers to hold on to, and some day she would greet her parents who had died when she was very young, when she got to heaven, just as her pastor had promised.

Mrs. Thomas is now faced with the decision as to how to respond to the news that she has cancer again. Her first husband would have wanted her to refuse the surgery because, once again, a blood transfusion would be needed. Her second husband, before his dementia, would have wanted her to do anything to stay alive. Her daughters became the voice of her first husband, and his son became the voice of her second husband.

Mrs. Thomas sought the assistance of the chaplain in the facility. She wanted help knowing what she ought to do. In her heart, she did not feel that surgery would do anything more than lower her own quality of life, even though she might live a bit longer. Not having surgery would allow her to follow the traditions of her first husband, yet his tradition would have allowed her to have chemotherapy, which she also felt would lower her quality of life. Somehow, she just wanted to be allowed to die in whatever way the natural course of the disease might take her, but she wanted to die with dignity.

Questions:
1. What influence did the three denominations play in Mrs. Thomas' final decision?
2. In what way did Mrs. Thomas' understanding of faith create conflict, while also sustaining her in her decision making?

Mrs. Thomas chose to do nothing, in defiance of both sides of the family. She lived quietly, in dignity for the next 6 months before she died in her apartment, with her daughters around her. At her request, her funeral was held in her childhood Baptist Church.

| CASE STUDY **2** | **Acting on Dreams** |

Objectives
1. Discuss the ways religion plays a part in pathology.
2. Examine religious dreams to determine if it is pathology or a mystical experience.
3. Understand how religion can be used in diagnosis.

Harold is 81 years old and white. He lives with his wife of 58 years in a small suburban home, and they have one son, who lives about 800 miles away. Harold has been a traveling salesman all of his life. He has not seen a physician in more than 5 years. For the past 20 years, his wife reports that when he needs medical assistance, he goes to a local clinic and generally sees a different doctor every time. All his life, Harold reports that he feels terrific sometimes and poorly at others. Generally, he feels good for a couple of weeks or a month and then feels poorly for a similar period of time.

Recently Harold was feeling poorly, but while he was asleep he had a dream that God came to him and told him to take up his bed and walk. When he woke up, he was feeling very good. He ran into his wife's bedroom and announced that God had told him to take up his bed and that was just what he planned to do and that he was starting right now. He got dressed and left the house. He arrived at his Presbyterian Church on foot just as the doors of the church were being opened for the day. He walked directly into the pastor's office and announced that God had told him to take up his bed and walk, so he has. He also noted that all of his friends had either died or moved to a warmer climate, so he needed to make new friends and wanted to start with the pastor. They talked for a time. The pastor noted that Harold seemed to talk very fast at times and at other times he seemed calmer. Although Harold had been a member of this church for the last 40 years, he had grown up Roman Catholic. He had started coming to this church because his wife was Presbyterian. He seemed to want to talk about what Presbyterians believed about heaven and hell, but he seemed to constantly distract himself from the discussion. He promised to be back to see the pastor, and he returned each morning for the next week.

At the end of the week, Harold reported to the pastor that his wife seemed to be unable to see when she woke up that morning. Harold was not sure what to do. The pastor worked with Harold to get his wife to the doctor. Betty was hospitalized and received numerous tests. However, no medical cause was ever found for her loss of vision. So she returned home, without her sight. This annoyed Harold a great deal, but he seemed to adjust. Betty seemed to want to sleep a lot, so Harold would leave her alone and call a taxi to go to the mall or to just go "do things."

The next Sunday was communion Sunday at the Presbyterian Church. (This church celebrates communion once a month). Harold and Betty arrived and sat in the front row of the church. This particular church uses a real loaf of bread and real wine as the elements for their communion service. When the bread was passed, Harold gave a piece to Betty and then took a second small piece, placed the piece back on the communion plate and passed the plate, proceeding to munch on the loaf for the remainder of the church service.

Harold continued to feel really good for the next month. During this time, he purchased a riding lawn mower with headlights; this way, he did not have to waste his time during the day mowing, he could mow after dark, often after midnight. He also went on a purchasing spree, buying things for the house such as furniture and other items that did not seem to be needed. This often made it hazardous for Betty to get around because Harold often left items in the living room without telling her about them.

At the end of the month, Harold reported that he had a visit from some of the older adults in the church. They wanted to talk with him about how he took communion. He reported that one of them also tried to tell him that he should do something more to help his wife with her blindness. That night Harold had another dream. He understood that God told him that his wife's blindness was the result of something he was doing, and with that he became very sad. He stopped going to see the pastor and attending church. His wife called the local Catholic Church on his behalf and requested a visit from a priest for last rites. Her vision seemed to be improving, so she cared for Harold until their son came and moved them both into a nursing home.

Harold was bipolar, probably for his entire life. His son reported that he was not aware of his father ever having been diagnosed with this disorder, but the behavior had existed for as long as he was aware.

His mother found Harold's constant mood swings extremely stressful, more so as she got older, leading to this instance of hysterical blindness. Harold lived for about 2 months in the nursing home and died of a sudden heart attack.

Questions:

1. How would you understand the dreams that Harold was having?
2. How can his interaction with the pastor help in diagnosis?
3. How could his church have played a more important role in helping Harold and Betty?

Rev. James W. Ellor, Ph.D., D. Min., LCSW, ACSW, BCD, DCSW, CGP, CSW-G
James Oberle, Ph.D.

References

Kosmin BA, Mayer E, Keysar A. *American Religious Identification Survey*. 46. New York: University of New York, 2001.

Nuland S. *How We Die*. New York: Alfred Knopf, 1994.

Robinson BA. Christian Meta-Groups: One Method of Sorting the Thousands of Christian Denominations into Groups. In: Ontario Consultants on Religious Tolerance; 2003. www.religioustolerance.org/chr_meta.htm (accessed April 2007).

Sullins DP. An organizational classification of Protestant denominations. *Rev Relig Res* 2004;45(3): 278–292.

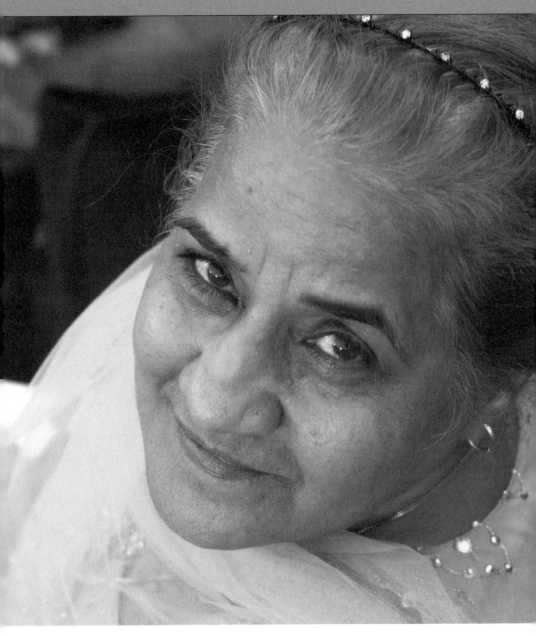

CHAPTER 5

Hinduism

About 900 million of the 6.5 billion world population are Hindus, making Hinduism the fourth largest religion in the world. The Hindu population in the United States is growing rapidly, from an estimated 227,000 in 1990 to an estimated 766,000 in 2001. Current estimates range from 1.1 to 1.5 million. Most US Hindus are either first-, second-, or third-generation immigrants with their religious and cultural practices of Hinduism greatly influenced by their country of origin (see table) and their level of acculturation.

Country	Estimate of Total Population, Hindu and non-Hindu	Percentage Hindu
India	1.03 billion[a]	80.5%
Nepal*	28,287,147[a]	80.6%
Bangladesh	147,365,352[b]	16%
UK	60,609,153[b]	1%
Mauritius	1,240,827[b]	48%
Sri Lanka	20,222,240[a]	7.1%

*Only official Hindu state in the world

[a]2001 census

[b]July 2006 estimate

Source: https://cia.gov/cia/publications/factbook/geos/xx.html (accessed April 2007).

Preferred Cultural Terms

> *Hinduism is one of the oldest organized religions in the world, tracing its roots back to 5000 BCE.*

The correct name of this ancient religion is "Sanatana Dharma," which means "eternal law" in Sanskrit. Also known as the Hindu Dharma, Hinduism is one of the oldest organized religions in the world, tracing its roots back to 5000 BCE. It originated in the Indian subcontinent on the banks of the Sindhu river (now Indus river) and was practiced by the Sindus (people who lived on the banks of the Sindhu), who were later known to the Greeks as Sindhus and finally as Hindus (a Persian word).

Philosophy and Scriptures

In contrast to some of the other organized religions, Hinduism can be more aptly described as a philosophy or way of life that has been subject to numerous interpretations over several millennia, now resulting in a religious practice that incorporates a remarkable diversity of cultural rituals and customs. Hinduism's philosophical core is rooted for the most part in the three fundamental Hindu scriptures: the *Vedas*, the *Upanishads*, and the *Bhagvad Gita*. Since Hinduism's inception over 5000 years ago, countless interpretations and reinterpretations of the sacred texts have obscured the line between religion and cultural practice. However, the philosophical tenets have remained remarkably constant.

According to the Hindu scriptures, the universe is believed to be unified by an all-pervasive power known as *Brahman* (not to be confused with *Brahmin*, a stratum of the outmoded Indian caste system). Hinduism states that the manifestation of the *Brahman* in living beings is the *Atman*, or soul, which is obscured from human awareness by layers of ignorance (*Agyana*). People, when in a state of *agyana*, are thought to be unaware of their fundamental unity with the universe. The goal for a Hindu is to pursue a path of righteous action, or *dharma*, that will eventually help shed these layers of ignorance and lead to *Moksha*, or ultimate enlightenment (the point at which the *Atman* unites with *Brahman*). These key principles are stated as *"Aham Bramhosmi"* (I am Brahman) and *"Tat Tuam Asi"* (You are It).

> *Hinduism is probably best described as a "polytheistic pantheism."*

Hinduism is probably best described as a "polytheistic pantheism." To a Hindu, the one God (*Brahman*) is eminent in the Universe and all pervasive. Everything is *Brahman,* and *Brahman* is everywhere. Hence, individuals have the freedom to worship the abstract, formless *Brahman* in any shape or form they choose (*Ishta Devatha*), thus leading to various manifestations of gods and goddesses who are thought to make up the Hindu pantheon. Some examples are the Hindu Trinity of Gods: namely *Brahma* the creator (not to be confused with *Brahman* the Supreme God), *Vishnu* the preserver, and *Shiva* the destroyer.

> *Karma is determined by a universal law (or order) in which good actions produce good results and bad actions produce bad results.*

The intent behind the apparent polytheism is to allow for Hinduism's complex philosophies to be more attainable to individuals. This freedom to worship the *Brahma* in *any* desired shape or form has also led to the Western misperceptions about the Hindu "Monkey God" and "Elephant God" (as described above, a Hindu is free to worship Brahman through any desired form), leading to cultural *faux pas.*

The pursuit and practice of the Hindu *dharma* is governed by a belief in *karma* (from the Sanskrit root "*kri,*" meaning "action")—the concept that every action leaves an imprint on one's *Atman. Karma* is determined by a universal law (or order) in which good actions produce good results and bad actions produce bad results. *Karmic* theory greatly influences the patient's world view of health, death, and dying and of the Hindu's explanatory model of illness. Furthermore, the results of *karma* can become manifest in a short timeframe or in the same lifetime, or they can carry over from previous lives or to future lives through rebirth.

Many Hindus may believe that pain and suffering (both physical and psychosocial) are the result of bad *karma* and not of medical or mental illness. Additionally, the *Atman* is immortal, and hence, most Hindus believe that the *Atman* must go through many lives until the aggregated good *karma* helps shed layers of ignorance that prevent the *Atman* from realizing its true nature and its ultimate goal of uniting with the *Brahman.* A common way of conceptualizing this is comparing the body to an article of clothing. The soul inhabits the body for as long as it can be useful and then casts it off in favor of a new body (garment). Thus for many Hindu patients, this life is not finite, and death is considered a transition point for the *Atman* (rather than a final end point), which will

> *For many Hindu patients, this life is not finite, and death is considered a transition point for the* Atman *(rather than a final end point).*

(depending on its accrued *karma*) either be repeatedly reborn in a new body or be united with the *Brahman*.

Older and more traditional Hindu adults may believe their illness is caused by bad *karma* from a past life or by past actions in this lifetime, and they may not entirely believe in the organic etiology propounded by Western biomedicine. As a result, an illness may be viewed as something to be accepted and endured rather than fixed or cured. In some situations, these beliefs may induce a quiet fatalism that can result in therapeutic nonadherence.

Formality of Address

The concept of respect is an important one for most traditional Hindus. Old age is often synonymous with wisdom, and the concepts of filial piety and ancestral worship are still very central to the practice of this ancient religion. Hindu elders often expect respectful and deferential treatment as their due. The term *"ji"* (for both men and women) or *"da"* (for men) is added to the end of a person's name or title to indicate respect (eg, Anita-*ji* or Basu-*da*). In turn, older Hindu adults often treat the physician with respect and deference and try their best (within their principles) to adhere to the physician's recommendations. Providers should address patients with warmth and respect and use a formal mode of address until given permission to use their first names, if ever. Younger and acculturated Hindus may be more willing to practice modern informality, but this should be determined by patient choice.

> *Older Hindu adults often treat the physician with respect and deference and try their best (within their principles) to adhere to the physician's recommendations.*

Language and Literacy

Most Asian Indian immigrants are well educated (85% are high school graduates, and more than 65% have college degrees), and many are well-qualified professionals (43% have graduate or professional degrees). About 80% of these Asian Indian immigrants practice Hinduism.

Respectful Nonverbal Communication

Older Hindu immigrants may be more accustomed to a paternalistic medical system in which the physician determines the care plan and makes the decisions. This premise does not apply to younger Hindu immigrants and more acculturated second- and third-generation Hindu Americans, who are more familiar with the patient-centered, customer-oriented model of modern biomedicine. An approach that works well with all Hindu Americans is using a tenor that is warm, respectful, and assured, and then tailoring specifics to suit the decision-making styles of individual patients and families. This approach is appropriate for both older adults who may still prefer the physician to make important decisions and for the younger generations who may prefer to take charge of their care plan. In regards to communication about health issues, most Hindus prefer a family-centered approach. Older adults and their children often prefer not to disclose negative information to patients because they worry that the truth may take away hope and increase suffering.

Older adults and their children often prefer not to disclose negative information to patients because they worry that the truth may take away hope and increase suffering.

Patterns of Immigration

Most Hindus living in the United States are of Asian Indian origin. Asian Indians came to the United States as early as 1790. However, the population did not grow significantly until passage of the Immigration and Naturalization Act of 1965, which opened the doors for individuals of certain professional or educational backgrounds. Hence, the 1960s cohort of Asian Indians who immigrated to the United States was a very highly educated and skilled group. Thereafter, laws were passed that allowed families to be reunited, and the Asian Indian population grew steadily through the 1970s and 1980s until a second spurt in the 1990s, heralded by the information technology boom.

Degree of Acculturation

According to the most recent census, approximately 1.7 million Asian Indians live in the United States, 80% being Hindus. An estimated 66,834 older Asian Indian adults live in the United States, most of whom are foreign born with an estimated 48,000 Hindu immigrant elders. The older Hindu immigrant population can be categorized into two major groups: those that immigrated around 1965 and have since settled in the United States and those who have come to live with their adult children who have immigrated to the United States. These two groups differ greatly demographically and face different issues. The former tend to be more acculturated, affluent, and independent. Those in the latter group are at high risk of being isolated and lonely (language barriers, lack of independent transportation), lack health benefits, depend on their children or family, and suffer from culture shock.

Tradition and Health Beliefs

Health care providers should be aware of some of the following customs and beliefs because it would help them provide culturally appropriate care—with the caveat that there is tremendous diversity in the Asian Indian Hindu population in the United States. Older Hindus who immigrated to the United States late in life may still be wedded to traditional Indian healing sciences of Ayurveda and Siddha.

> Ayurveda is an ancient and sophisticated healing art that originated in the Indian subcontinent.

Ayurveda is an ancient and sophisticated healing art that originated in the Indian subcontinent. It is a comprehensive and holistic healing art thought to have been derived from the *Atharveda,* one of the oldest Hindu scriptures. It dates back to 1000 BCE and includes both herbal remedies and surgical techniques *(salya-chikitsa)* aimed at preserving life *(ayus)* and promoting well-being. Practitioners used mercury- and sulfur-based medications and herbs to treat ailments and emetic herbs to maintain body homeostasis or balance of the *tridosha* (three humoral systems): *pitha* (fire), *vatha* (wind), and *kapha* (water).

Siddha uses calcinated metals and mineral powders to heal illnesses.

Clinicians should use a gentle and nonjudgmental manner to ask about these healing systems and then document use of herbs or complementary and alternative medications. It is also important to educate patients about any potential drug-herb interactions if the patient is concurrently using Western medications as well.

> Older Hindus often practice regular upwas or fasts during which they may not eat or drink for extended periods.

Other Hindu and Cultural Beliefs and Rituals

Upwas

Older Hindus often practice regular *upwas* or fasts during which they may not eat or drink for extended periods. This may be done regularly (weekly, monthly, etc), and strict practitioners may not take their medications during a religious fast. In some cases, older patients may take their medications during *upwas* but refuse to take any food or fluids. This can be problematic in diabetic patients who may be taking their antiglycemic medications during *upwas* days but not food, or taking neither food nor medication.

Muhurat

Certain days of the month are thought to be auspicious times and days (based on the Hindu lunar calendar). Traditional Hindu Americans may request that elective surgical procedures (eg, hip replacements) be performed on these days.

Raahukala and Yamakanda

These are particular 90-minute periods within a day when older Hindu adults may be reluctant to undertake important actions (such as a medical visit). Patients may worry that taking actions during these inauspicious time periods will have a negative impact on the outcome.

Religious Paraphernalia

Married Indian women often wear the *Mangalsutra*, a sacred necklace, around their necks. Hindu men wear the *Upanayanam Poonal* sacred thread around their torso. These items are considered sacred and important and should never be cut or removed without the explicit consent of the patient or family. Ritualistic wrist or waist bands also should be considered sacred. Hindu women often wear a *tikka* (dot on the forehead) or *Sindur* (red pigment on the hairline). When asked to remove these religious paraphernalia as a part of preoperative preparation, some patients may offer resistance. If resistance continues after the patient and family have been educated about the need for a sterile field in surgical procedures, the patient should be allowed to retain these items but requested to sign an informed consent form about the risk of infection.

Stigma Associated with Mental Illness

Mental illness is often considered a taboo, especially among the older Hindu population. *Dil udhas hona* is the term for "the blues" or depression in the Hindi, Urdu, Punjabi, and Gujarati languages. Traditional older Hindus may be resistant to admitting experiencing symptoms of any mental illness such as depression. They may refuse

Traditional older Hindus may be resistant to admitting experiencing symptoms of any mental illness such as depression.

to believe that depression is an organic syndrome and that it can be treated with medications. In contrast, they may believe that feelings of sadness or hopelessness are a result of past *karma* and that the illness-associated suffering will eventually wash away the *karma* and, thus, should not be palliated with medications.

Culture-Specific Health Risks

Consanguinity

Marrying the offspring of a mother's brother or a father's sister is an acceptable traditional practice, but marrying the offspring of a mother's sister or a father's brother is not. Although this is falling out of favor as the medical risks associated with consanguinity are better understood, older Hindus may be offspring of a consanguineous marriage.

Dietary Practices

Rice remains a dietary staple for Hindus from Southern India, and wheat for those from Northern India. Many older Hindus are vegetarians or vegans. Chicken, mutton, and fish are consumed by Hindus who are not vegetarians. Traditional Hindus rarely eat beef. However, globalization and acculturation to American ways have had a strong influence on Hindu dietary habits. Lactose intolerance is very common in older Asian Indians. The Hindu diet is rich in carbohydrates, poor in protein, and often deficient in calcium. Thus, older adults are at risk of protein calorie malnutrition and osteoporosis. Older Hindus may consume betel leaves (*Piper betel* Linn). Betel leaves, which are the main ingredients in *pan* or *tambool* that Hindus (especially married people) chew, are thought to be carminatives with antiflatulent and anti-inflammatory effects. In Ayurvedic medicine, betel leaves are used as an aphrodisiac. Many chew tobacco with betel leaves, which puts them at risk of oral submucosal fibrosis.

> *The Hindu diet is rich in carbohydrates, poor in protein, and often deficient in calcium.*

Hindu Americans are at high risk of insulin resistance leading to diabetes mellitus type 2, and dyslipidemia, which causes increased visceral adipose tissue and eventually coronary artery disease. This is further aided by the belief of the older Hindu generation that the 'Ghee' (pronounced "gē"), or clarified butter, strengthens the body and promotes good health. The prevalence of Alzheimer's disease is very low in India, but the predilection to diabetes and coronary artery disease increases the risk of multi-infarct dementia.

Approaches to Decision Making

Many traditional Hindu families have a hierarchy of decision makers in place, usually beginning with the oldest son as the primary contact and disseminator of information. Families may often consult physicians whom they know personally to get as much information as possible. This reflects a need to be well informed about the situation rather than a distrust of health care providers. Families may be reluctant to discuss personal, emotional, and financial issues with health care providers because these matters are considered very private and traditionally are not shared with anyone other than those in the immediate household.

> *Families may be reluctant to discuss personal, emotional, and financial issues with health care providers.*

Traditionally, Hindu society has been male dominated, with women assuming a submissive or passive role. In the modern era, the role of Hindu women is rapidly evolving. Many women play active roles in decision-making processes, although men may continue to serve as spokespersons of the family unit. Thus, clinicians should avoid stereotypical generalizations and ask open-ended questions to explore the values and decision-making styles of individual families.

Disclosure and Consent

Hindu families are interdependent with the autonomous unit consisting of the patient and spouse, adult children, and key members of the extended family. As described earlier, any health care professionals in the extended family are traditionally often called on to interpret test results and help with decision making.

Older adults who are ill may practice "closed awareness" (ie, although they may be fully aware of the gravity of their illness, they may be unwilling to openly discuss their illness and prognosis with their family). Similarly, family members may request that the physician withhold information from their loved one who is ill due to the concern that the truth about the illness may negate the will to live. Thus, *"Doctor saab (sir), please don't tell Dada-ji (grandfather) that he has cancer. He will just give up and die"* may not be an uncommon request from a Hindu American family.

> *Family members may request that the physician withhold information from their loved one who is ill due to the concern that the truth about the illness may negate the will to live.*

Gender Issues

The concept of shyness, or *shrm*, in women is thought to be feminine and thus much valued in traditional India. As a consequence, older Hindu women may be soft-spoken and unwilling to be asked or to answer frank questions about intimate behaviors and practices (eg, sexual history, incontinence, bowel regimens). They often prefer to be examined by same-sex health professionals, although more acculturated and younger Hindu women may be very similar to their Western counterparts. Sensitive inquiry will elicit most of the patient's preferences, and any sincere attempt to honor their preferences is greatly valued and appreciated. Having a female relative available when examining an older Hindu woman is a highly recommended practice because it facilitates a frank interaction.

> *Having a female relative available when examining an older Hindu woman is a highly recommended practice because it facilitates a frank interaction.*

End-of-Life Decision Making and Intensity of Care

Although very few studies have been conducted regarding the prevalence of and knowledge about advance care directives among Asian Indian Hindus, the data indicate that many individuals do not have these documents. This may hold particularly true for older Hindu adults who were born in India. Small studies have also shown an inverse relationship between the strength of religious and traditional beliefs and the presence of a completed advance care directive. As mentioned earlier, Hindu philosophy has a multitude of interpretations that have become intricately woven into cultural customs and traditions that vary tremendously among regions in India. Furthermore, Hindus may not view death as a final event but more as a transition for the soul from one life to the next. The family plays a central role at the time of terminal illness or death. From a traditional Hindu perspective, it is very important for the family members to be at the bedside of the terminally ill patient praying, chanting hymns, or bringing in pictures or idols of gods/goddesses, especially the Trinity and their spouses, viz, Vishnu and his consort Lashmi, Shiva and his consort Parvati, and less often Brahma and his consort Saraswathi. Some families may be hesitant to allow health care providers to give a dying patient sedating

> *Hindus may not view death as a final event but more as a transition for the soul from one life to the next.*

medications (because it may be important to the family that the patient be as awake as possible through the dying process). These traditions reflect a belief that dying individuals should be thinking of God as they go through the dying process, because it is believed that the nature of one's thoughts at the time of death determines the destination of the departing soul. However, if the clinician identifies that the patient is experiencing intractable suffering caused by refractory symptoms (eg, pain or dyspnea) and is requesting palliation of these symptoms, sedation of the patient and gentle education of the family members will likely result in assent with needed palliative measures.

At the time of death, family members may request that the body be positioned in specific directions (head facing east for some and feet facing south for others) or that it be placed on the ground (return to mother earth). Families may also request that providers allow them to place a *Tulsi* (*Ocimum Sanctum*) leaf or drops of water from the Ganga River on a patient's lips. Again, this allows a patient to focus on God as their soul leaves the body.

After death, it may be important for family members (of the same gender) to be allowed to perform ritual washing of the body and prepare it for cremation (typically Hindus do not bury their dead), which should ideally be done within 24 hours of death. Most Hindu families will not request an autopsy but may not be opposed if there are clear reasons for it. Regardless, this is a delicate topic and should be approached with the sensitivity it deserves.

> *Most Hindu families will not request an autopsy but may not be opposed if there are clear reasons for it.*

CASE STUDY **1**	**Palliative Care and Family Decisions**

Objectives
1. Highlight some traditional approaches to medical decision making of older Hindu adults and their families.
2. Understand some important perspectives of older Hindu adults toward the management of terminal illnesses.
3. Realize potential areas of conflict between wishes of terminally ill older Hindu adults and their families and standards of practice in Western hospitals.

Mrs. Prasad is a 78-year-old Asian Indian woman with an extensive history of hypertension, diabetes, and hyperlipidemia. She has recently arrived from India to live with her children after her husband passed away. Although her family believes that her medical problems are under control because she was being cared for by a doctor in India, she has not told anyone that she has been experiencing chest tightness and some shortness of breath when she walks or exerts herself. Furthermore, she has not told her family that she does not regularly take her diabetes medications, preferring to control her blood sugar with specific foods and fasts that her friends have told her about.

One morning, while eating breakfast, she develops severe crushing chest pain and cannot breathe properly. Her family rushes her to the local emergency department, and she arrives accompanied by her son, daughter-in-law, and two young grandchildren. Soon after, her daughter comes to the hospital as well. Initial diagnostic studies reveal that she has had a massive acute ST elevation anterolateral myocardial infarction. The cardiology team has come to evaluate the patient, and key decisions need to be made regarding her plan of care.

Questions:
1. What important customs, beliefs, and communication styles common to many older Hindu adults have to be considered in the events predating Mrs. Prasad's heart attack?
2. How should the cardiology team approach the urgent discussions regarding the plan for her care?

The decision is made to take Mrs. Prasad to the cardiac catheterization laboratory, where severe triple vessel disease is discovered. The cardiac surgeons are consulted and Mrs. Prasad undergoes a coronary artery bypass graft. During the surgery, her vessels are noted to be small and tortuous, but the surgeon has had experience operating on Asian Indians and feels that the procedure goes well overall. She is then transferred from the recovery room to the intensive care unit and intubated. She is on a variety of medications to stabilize her condition.

Over the next several days, Mrs. Prasad's condition remains critical. She has episodes of atrial fibrillation, heart failure, and delirium, and she remains dependent on the mechanical ventilator. Ongoing discussions are held between family members and the health care team regarding her condition. Although Mrs. Prasad had not completed any advance care directives before this illness, it becomes clear that she had expressed her wishes regarding aggressive care at this stage of her life to her children.

Approximately 1 week after the coronary artery bypass graft, Mrs. Prasad starts to have high fevers, and the nursing staff notes she has thick secretions in her endotracheal tube. She is started on broad-spectrum antibiotics for a nosocomial pneumonia, but her condition continues to decline. She has several episodes of heart failure thought to be due to intermittent hypoxemia, and her renal function has started to deteriorate. Three days after starting the antibiotics, Mrs. Prasad develops profound hypotension and renal failure necessitating treatment with pressors. Her renal failure is now worse and the team feels that she will need continuous venovenous hemodialysis in light of her unstable state.

Discussions are held with the family, and they understand Mrs. Prasad's serious state. A decision is made not to start hemodialysis and to pursue comfort measures only at this point with the understanding that Mrs. Prasad will likely pass away.

Questions:

1. When an older Hindu adult is diagnosed with a terminal condition or serious illness, what concepts from Hinduism may influence decisions about treatment?
2. What aspects of comfort care can be difficult for Hindu patients and their families to accept? How might one assist the family in making this transition?

Mrs. Prasad is not started on dialysis, and the antibiotics are stopped. Although she is intermittently awake, she has more periods of lethargy and somnolence. Her blood pressure remains very low despite the use of pressors, and she remains febrile although periodic acetaminophen, administered through her nasogastric tube, provides relief. She does not seem to be in any pain. As Mrs. Prasad begins the dying process, the nursing staff is overwhelmed by the turnout of family and friends who are at the patient's bedside whenever visiting hours allow. They are bewildered by the constant requests to have religious songs played at all times for the patient and by the placement of pictures and small idols of different deities around the room. One nurse had to warn a family member to not put any water or item near the patient's mouth, because she was *npo*. Mrs. Prasad seems comfortable, but her family is very upset that she is being allowed to die in such a manner. They request a meeting with the patient services representative, which leads to a larger family meeting with the health care team and the family. By the time Mrs. Prasad passes away, the family and the staff feel better. The family denies a request for an autopsy, and Mrs. Prasad is cremated the next day according to the family's wishes.

Questions:

1. What important customs and rituals related to death and dying for a Hindu adult may be at conflict with traditional care practices in a hospital or institution?
2. What are some ways to accommodate important aspects of care for both parties involved?

CASE STUDY **2**	**The Cultural Influence on Perception of Mental Illness**

Objectives
1. Understand the importance of travel and immigration history and its impact on health of older immigrant adults.
2. Realize that mental illness might be associated with great stigma in certain cultures and understand the need to approach this topic with the sensitivity it requires.

Mr. Rajan Sharma is an 80-year-old Hindu American immigrant with a medical history of diabetes mellitus that is controlled by diet. Last week, he was admitted to the hospital for shortness of breath and confusion. A month before admission, he was stable, ambulatory, and actively involved with the Sanatana Dharma Hindu Community Center, conducting Hindi classes for children. Two weeks before admission, his only son, Anand (patient lives with his son's family), had noticed that his father had become progressively more tired and on some days remained in bed until noon. Anand was disturbed by this new change in his father's routine because Mr. Sharma had prided himself all his life on waking up at five o'clock every morning and performing the Hindu ceremonial *pooja* (prayer) for over 2 hours. A week before admission, Anand's wife noticed that her father-in-law was not eating well and seemed to "be ill." Three days before admission, Mr. Sharma became progressively weak and short of breath and was subsequently admitted to the hospital.

Mr. Sharma had worked for Bank of India and had lived in Pune, India, for several years after retirement. He and his wife had immigrated to the United States 7 years ago to be reunited with their only son. Mrs. Sharma died 8 months ago of "heart disease." Mr. Sharma had cremated his beloved wife of 59 years and had insisted on taking her remains back to India to dissolve the ashes in the Ganga River. Despite Anand's best efforts to dissuade him, Mr. Sharma had insisted on going alone, stating "a pious Hindu will never shirk his duty to his wife." He completed this arduous journey and returned 5 months ago, tired and desolate.

On clinical examination, the liver was enlarged (10 sonometers below the right costal margin), and breath sounds were decreased on the base of the right lung. A chest radiograph was consistent with right-sided pleural effusion, and abdominal ultrasonography revealed a large hepatic cyst. A right-sided thoracentesis produced "anchovy sauce pus." Mr. Sharma was diagnosed with amoebasis with amoebic liver abscess and amoebic pleural effusion. He had a protracted but mostly uneventful hospital course and was discharged to his son's home.

Questions:
1. Why is taking a detailed immigrant and travel history an important consideration when working with older immigrants?
2. Why is functional status thought to be an important assessment measure in providing care for older adults?

Two months after hospitalization, you see Mr. Sharma in your clinic. You note that he has recovered well from his amoebiasis and has been taking his medications very regularly. However, he has lost 9 pounds, and his current body mass index is 19. Furthermore, his daughter-in-law, Gowri (who has accompanied him to the clinic), reports that Mr. Sharma stays at home and has refused to return to the Sanatana Dharma Hindu Community Center or to participate in any social activities. He does play with his grandchildren but not as much as he used to. Gowri states that they tried some Ayurvedic tonics to improve his energy but without success. She requests "a powerful tonic or a vitamin" to make him feel better. On further questioning, Mr. Sharma states that he has trouble remembering and complains bitterly about his "memory failing him." He states that this is the main reason for discontinuing his community activities. You perform a Mini–Mental Status Examination (MMSE), and his score is 25/30. You tell Mr. Sharma and his daughter-in-law that you think he has dementia. Immediately, Mr. Sharma looks agitated and states loudly in Hindi *"Main paagal nahin"* (I am not mad) and angrily leaves the clinic. Gowri looks troubled and says "Sorry, doctor saab. I did not realize that mental illness ran in my husband's side of the family. I will have my husband bring his father back to see you."

Questions:
1. Given Mr. Sharma's recent history, what other screening and assessment tool might be appropriate along with an MMSE?
2. What are some considerations to be taken into account when discussing mental health issues with older Hindu adults and their families?

CASE STUDY **3**	**Providing Quality Health Care While Respecting Hindu Communication Traditions**

Objectives

1. Understand the balance between maintaining health status and respecting religious beliefs and practices of a Hindu immigrant.
2. Discuss ways to render health care without conflicting with lifelong social and moral principles of an older Hindu immigrant.

You are a primary care physician in a small town at the outskirts of a metropolitan area. Besides providing primary care, you are also in charge of a four-bed intensive care unit at the small local hospital. You are requested to see a new patient, Mrs. Savita. She is 76 years old and has recently come from India to live with her son, Raj, who recently joined the local hospital to manage its IT department. Although Raj is delighted to have his mother with him because it provides an opportunity to serve her and fulfill his duties as a son, he is also worried about her health. His wife, Lakshmi, is also expecting their first child and is due in the next few weeks. Between the pressures of his new job, his wife's condition, and his mother's health status, Raj is very concerned. Given your reputation as an excellent physician, Raj is looking to you with great hopes. Mrs. Savita is obese, pleasant, and very religious; she retired from a managerial job a few years ago. She has recently been complaining of fatigue, weakness, blurry vision, and numbness in her hands and feet. She had lost noticeable weight about a month ago but is now eating a lot and has almost gained it back. She also drinks a lot of water and wakes up several times a night to urinate. She feels sad sometimes and sits quietly, yet at other times becomes upset over minor issues. These problems were initially ignored as adjustment issues to the new culture. Mrs. Savita thinks that there is something wrong because she has never had these problems before. She thinks that God is punishing her for something that she has done wrong in the past.

Questions:

1. What is your opinion about Mrs. Savita's condition? Do you think there is something wrong medically, or is it a social adjustment issue in the new environment?

2. What is your opinion about Mrs. Savita's views that the God is punishing her for her past deeds?

You examine Mrs. Savita and find nothing wrong except paresthesias on the dorsum of both her forearm and the right leg. You order routine laboratory tests. It is a Monday, and because Mrs. Savita fasts every Monday, the blood samples are fasting. The blood glucose concentration is 280 mg%. The urine shows traces of sugar but no ketones. You call Mrs. Savita and suggest repeating the fasting blood glucose concentration next morning. The result is 276 mg%. Raj sees you at the hospital and asks for the results. He is very anxious to know why the test was repeated. Because he is the next of kin of the patient, you tell him the results and that his mother has diabetes mellitus. Raj's face drops, and he says that his maternal grandfather and a maternal uncle both had diabetes and died relatively young. He requests you not tell his mother about the diagnosis because she thinks it is a deadly disease. You ask him to bring his mother to the clinic the next day for further management. When Mrs. Savita arrives the next day with her son, you discuss the test results in a nonspecific manner and ask Mrs. Savita if she would like you to discuss her health issues directly or with someone else to act on her behalf and make health care decisions. She tells you that because she does not know anything about this new place, she would rather trust her son, who has been living here for 5 years, to make decisions for her. She just wants to feel better.

Questions:

1. Knowing the HIPAA regulations and the fact that Raj is a fellow employee and his mother is dependent on him, how comfortable did you feel discussing Mrs. Savita's test results with him? Did you notice any culture-specific value when Raj requested that you not give his mother the diagnosis per se?

2. You dealt with the patient autonomy issue by bringing up the issue of health care decision making earlier in your encounter. Weren't you relieved?

Sensing the strong dynamics between the mother and the son and feeling a bit relieved that you saved Mrs. Savita from the emotional trauma of knowing her specific diagnosis, you start her on a diabetic diet and suggest weight reduction and exercise. You also suggest increased social activities to give Mrs. Savita more exposure to the local culture. Raj smiles, and both mother and son leave, thanking you for your help.

Question:

1. As a native-born American and a physician who grew up in Western culture and trained in Western medicine, how do you feel about the whole encounter? Did your view that the diseases are a result of pathologic processes rather than past deeds strike you anytime during the encounter?

A few weeks later, you receive a frantic call from Raj saying that his mother is not feeling well. She is complaining of abdominal pain, has vomited a few times, and is very weak and lethargic. She is also acting strangely, stating that "God is punishing me" and sometimes "I am Goddess Kali, I will rid this earth of demons." On further inquiry, he tells you that his mother has been observing *Navratra* for the last 8 days, a religious period of fasting for 9 days, during which some people do not eat or drink anything, while some eat a miniscule amount of dairy or vegetarian food. Thinking that something serious is going on, you ask him to bring his mother to the hospital at once. When she arrives, she appears dehydrated with dry skin and tongue and a tender abdomen without rebound tenderness. She is afebrile with a regular pulse of 88 per minute, blood pressure of 148/76 mmHg, and a respiratory rate of 36 per minute. Laboratory tests have the following results: serum glucose 586 mg%, serum sodium 149 mEq/L, potassium 5.8 mEq/L, chloride 110 mEq/L, bicarbonate 6 mEq/L, BUN 56 mg%, creatinine 2.3%, and pH 7.162.

Questions:

1. What do you think about the course of events? What is your opinion about Mrs. Savita fasting every Monday and this prolonged fast of 9 days, in spite of her being a diabetic patient?
2. Mrs. Savita thinks that the God is punishing her for her past deeds in the form of her current ailment. How would you deal with this?

You diagnose Mrs. Savita as having diabetic ketoacidosis. You admit her to the intensive care unit and start her on intravenous fluid and insulin infusion and monitor her electrolytes, blood glucose, serum insulin level, and blood gases. The next day, when her acidosis has cleared and bicarbonate concentration is normal, you stop this treatment and start feeding. Because the ninth day of fasting had passed, she accepts the food and is on her road to recovery.

Perplexed by the sequence of events, you call a meeting with Mrs. Savita and Raj. Respecting the wishes expressed previously, you emphasize the importance of maintaining a caloric balance and proper hydration, without explicitly referring to the diagnosis per se. You also discuss alternatives in a situation like this. Raj states that when his mother is fasting, she will not accept anything that is considered a food but may still accept substances considered medicines. This appeared to be a great suggestion and led to formulating a plan to maintain fluid and caloric balance during fasting. Armed with the plan and relieved that they can better deal with such situations in the future, both Mrs. Savita and Raj left your office, marveling about your great professional acumen.

VS Periyakoil, MD

AR Rao, MD

P Sharma, MD

References

Barnes JS, Bennett CF. The Asian population; 2000. Available at: www.census.gov/prod/2002pubs/c2kbr01-16.pdf (accessed December 2007).

Bhagavad Gita Translated for Modern Readers. Tomales, CA: Niligiri Press; 1985 (trans. Easwaran E).

Bhungalia S, Kemp C. (Asian) Indian health beliefs and practices related to the end of life. *J Hosp Palliat Nurs* 2002;4:54–58.

Deshpande O, Reid MC, Rao AS. Attitudes of Asian-Indian Hindus toward end-of-life care. *J Am Geriatr Soc* 2005;53:131–135.

Doorenbos AZ, Nies MA. The use of advance directives in a population of Asian Indian Hindus. *J Transcult Nurs* 2003;14:17–24.

http://fpc.state.gov/documents/organization/80669.pdf (accessed May 2007).

https://cia.gov/cia/publications/factbook/geos/xx.html (accessed April, 2007).

Ivey SL, Patel S, Kalra P, Greenlund K, Srinivasan S, Grewal D. Cardiovascular health among Asian Indians (CHAI): A community research project. *J Interprofess Care* 2004;18(4):391–402.

Jensen JM. *Passage from India: Asian Indian Immigrants in North America.* New Haven, CT: Yale University Press; 1988.

Kosmin BA, Mayer E. Religious identification study, 2001. Available at: http://www.gc.cuny.edu/faculty/research_briefs/aris/aris_index.htm (accessed April 2007).

Laungani P. Hindu deaths in India—Part 1. *Int J Health Prom Educ* 2001;39:114–120.

Pandit B. *Hindu Dharma.* Glen Ellyn, IL: BV Enterprises; 1996.

Periyakoil V. Older Asian Indian Americans. In: Adler R, Kamel H (eds). *Doorway Thoughts: Cross-Cultural Health Care for Older Adults.* Sudbury, MA: Jones & Bartlett/American Geriatrics Society; 2004.

Shaji S, Bose S, Verghese A. Prevalence of dementia in an urban population in Kerala, India. *Brit J Psychol* 2005;186:136–140.

Smith H. *The World's Religions*. San Francisco: Harper; 1991:64.

Upanishads. New York: Oxford University Press; 1996 (trans. Olivell P). www.census.gov/ (accessed May 2007).

CHAPTER 6

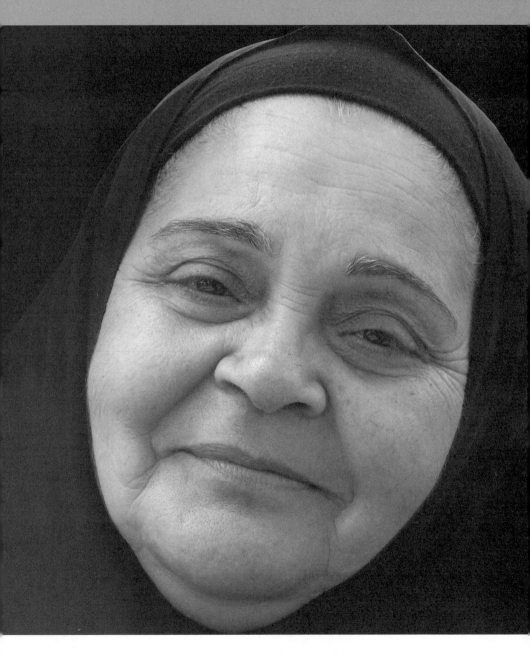

Islam

Islam is a monotheistic religion that considers itself a continuation of God's revelations to humanity concerning their existence and relationship with Him. A Muslim believes in the absolute oneness and unity of God (*Allah* in Arabic) and in the Prophethood of Muhammad, who conveyed the final message of God to humankind. Muslims view life as a test for human beings, who are granted free will, ie, the capacity to choose with full responsibility and accountability for one's choices; hence, the Islamic belief in the Day of Judgment.

Muslims view life as a test for human beings, who are granted free will.

Muslims in the United States come from diverse cultural, social, economic, and educational backgrounds that inform, sometimes to a larger degree than the Islamic tradition, the way they act and behave. Islam has a long history of pluralism manifested in its sects and schools of jurisprudence. The level of an individual's adherence to Islamic teachings also creates diversity among Muslims. The culturally and spiritually astute clinician will bear all these factors in mind when interacting with any individual patient and understanding his or her unique cultural and spiritual practices.

Diversity Among Muslims

There are approximately 6–7 million Muslims in the United States; 32% of American Muslims are South Asian, 26% Arabs, 20% African American, 7% African, and 15% representing various other ethnicities. There is no typical look or appearance of a Muslim. American Muslims represent all cultures, ethnic, and national backgrounds, and all sects of the world Muslim communities.

American Muslims represent all cultures, ethnic, and national backgrounds, and all sects of the world Muslim communities.

There are two major sects within the Muslim community: Sunnis represent 80%–85% of the total Muslim world population, while Shiites represent 15%–20%. Counsel for Muslim patients should be sought from their co-sectarian religious authority when available.

Some older Muslims may also keep a small copy of the Qur'an or a small booklet of invocations close at hand or attached to their bodies.

Holy Texts

The two main sources of guidance for Muslims are the *Qur'an*, held by Muslims to be God's direct revelation to the Prophet Muhammad, and the *Sunnah*, the normative sayings and deeds of Prophet Muhammad. In addition to seeking biomedical cures, many older Muslims recite verses from the Qur'an and key invocations from both the Qur'an and the Sunnah as crucial elements in the healing process. Reverence and total silence on the part of the listeners accompany such recitation. Some older Muslims may also keep a small copy of the Qur'an or a small booklet of invocations close at hand or attached to their bodies. When possible, these objects should not be removed except with the explicit consent of the patient or a family member.

The religious Sabbath for Muslims falls on every Friday.

Important Holidays and Celebrations

The two cardinal holy days in Islam are Eid-ul-Adha, marking the completion of the annual pilgrimage to Mecca, Saudi Arabia, and Eid-ul-Fitr, celebrating the completion of fasting in the lunar month of Ramadan, the ninth month of the Islamic calendar. These are spiritually significant days for many Muslims. Many older Muslims will avoid scheduling surgery or appointments on these festivals. The religious Sabbath for Muslims falls on every Friday. During that time, many observant Muslim men attend Friday congregational prayer at the mosque and avoid scheduling appointments around noontime. Some Muslim women also attend prayer and may wish to delay appointments or elective procedures. Daily prayers have greater flexibility in their times than the Friday prayer. For many older Muslims, the Friday prayer also provides an avenue for social interaction with extended family and friends who share a similar cultural background. The inability to attend the Friday congregation is sometimes an important spiritual concern for patients (although they are exempt from attending), and involvement of a Muslim chaplain or spiritual leader might be needed.

Religious Basis for Views on Health and Illness

According to Islamic teachings, both health and illness are parts of the test of life. Health is considered a bounty from God, worthy of appreciation and protection. Preventive health should be emphasized to older Muslims. Showing compassion for and visiting the sick is another way that Muslims express their gratitude for their own health.

Showing compassion for and visiting the sick is another way that Muslims express their gratitude for their own health.

Sickness is also a test, although not necessarily of patients. For example, a child's illness is seen as a test for their parents, or even for the whole society, that is required to establish adequate health care resources. Seeking treatment for illness is religiously recommended, and some Muslim scholars consider it an obligation. The Islamic concept of suffering emphasizes that Divine justice will recompense, without measure, a person's suffering. While suffering is rewarded, however, so is seeking a cure, because it prolongs a person's ability to worship God and to do good for humankind. In summary, suffering is accepted, but a cure is desired. Some Muslims view illness as a punishment for their sins, for which feelings of guilt and despair can be overwhelming. In such cases, a Muslim spiritual adviser should be consulted.

Muslim Family Structure

In Islam, great emphasis is placed on support, solidarity, and continued care among family members. In many Muslim cultures, it is the norm for extended families to live together or within close proximity. This may not be possible in all cases among American Muslims because of immigration laws, and it is not the case with most Muslim converts. In most Muslim cultures, older Muslims enjoy much respect within their families and continue to live and receive care in their children's homes even after their children are married. In many Muslim cultures, not caring for the older Muslims in one's own home may be interpreted as abandonment. Such perception may bring shame and embarrassment, and lead to severance of family ties.

In many Muslim cultures, not caring for the older Muslims in one's own home may be interpreted as abandonment.

In the extended family structure, decisions about personal medical matters are not made by the concerned individuals alone, but rather by his or her family, including the spouse, siblings, parents, and children. This multigenerational decision making in Muslim families can pose a challenge for health care providers when, for example, they find themselves caught between the interests and concerns of the older and younger members of the family. One potentially helpful strategy in this situation would be for health care providers to identify common values that guide the behaviors of the older Muslim's family. For example, a question like, "What do you think your mother would like to be done for her?" might encourage the family to consider treatment options that are in the best interest of the patient, owing to their filial piety toward the older Muslim patient.

Cultural and Religious Practices that Affect the Health Care Setting

During life-threatening medical emergencies, everything should be done to save a life, and any of the religious practices discussed below can be temporarily suspended or postponed.

Gender Interaction

Modesty is an important concept in Islam. For men, modest dress entails covering the area between the navel to the knees, as well as the legs and often the upper arms. In dire circumstances, covering the genitals is a bare minimum unless it hinders life-saving medical care. For women, modesty entails covering the whole body except the face, the hands, and the feet. Older women are religiously exempt from adhering to some of these requirements. Culturally, some women may prefer to cover part or all of their face, while others may not adhere to such requirements regardless of age.

Modesty is an important concept in Islam.

Physical contact with the opposite sex should be limited to what is medically necessary. For example, health care providers should avoid shaking hands with a patient of the opposite sex unless the patient initiates the gesture. During physical examinations and nursing care, particularly for intimate care, same-sex practitioners should be called on whenever possible. If a same-sex practitioner is not available, a medical chaperone should be present. Exposure and touching should be limited to only those areas of the body that need medical attention. Some women may want to continue to wear their headscarf throughout their hospital stay except when bathing or in assured privacy. When possible,

Health care providers should avoid shaking hands with a patient of the opposite sex unless the patient initiates the gesture.

this wish should be respected. Direct eye contact between the opposite sexes is discouraged; it can be interpreted negatively and should be avoided or minimized.

Dietary Restrictions

Muslims do not eat pork or drink alcohol. Medicinal tinctures and elixirs made with alcohol are not permissible unless they are the sole or best form of a therapeutic preparation available. Porcine therapeutics and organs are allowed if they are the best form of treatment or necessary to save a life. Gelatin capsules and gelatin-containing foods are generally considered permissible independent of their source of production, although some Muslims object, regardless. Many Muslims insist on Zabihah meat (beef and poultry slaughtered by Muslims in a ritual fashion). Seafood is acceptable, except shrimp and shellfish, which some Muslims find objectionable. The older Muslim's individual preferences should be assessed to ensure compliance with his or her religious and personal dietary preferences.

Rituals that Affect Health Care

Islamic rituals of worship create a rhythm in a Muslim's life. Muslim patients may wish to maintain this rhythm, despite their illness and hospitalization.

Prayer: Islamic prayer consists of ritualized movements and recitations that involve standing, sitting, genuflecting, and prostrating oneself. The prayers are timed for specific intervals of the day. If possible, arranging medical examinations and procedures around the prayer time is preferred; otherwise, informing a Muslim patient of scheduled diagnostic tests or therapy sessions is helpful to allow the patient to plan prayers accordingly.

Islamic prayer consists of ritualized movements and recitations that involve standing, sitting, genuflecting, and prostrating oneself.

Ambulatory inpatients often prefer a chapel to pray in and appreciate having portable oxygen available and their intravenous line "locked" for greater mobility. Those who cannot leave their room may prefer a blanket or other clean item to place on the floor during prostration. Those who cannot leave their bed will pray in place. The casual observer may think such patients are having a stroke because they will appear to be whispering to themselves, engaged in strange repetitive movements, remaining unresponsive to queries or conversation. Therefore, it is important to understand when a Muslim patient may be praying.

Most Muslim scholars agree that any part of the body that may be harmed by water during ablutions can be overlooked.

Ablution: The ritual washings that precede prayer require wetting the arms and feet, where intravenous catheters are often placed, with water. Most Muslim scholars agree that any part of the body that may be harmed by water during ablutions can be overlooked. However, some Muslims may wish to wet the area around the catheter or remove the tape. In this case, the necessity of the catheter and securing tape can be explained to avoid confusion (excessive tape should be avoided during application).

Fasting: Fasting from dawn to sunset during the month of Ramadan is one of the pillars of Islam. The fast involves complete abstinence from ingesting any substance (nutritive or non-nutritive), including oral medication. Some scholars allow nebulized and injected medications, such as albuterol and insulin, while others do not. Older Muslims with a weak constitution, or any Muslim adult who is ill from an acute, chronic, or incurable disease, are exempt from fasting. However, some Muslims wish to fast regardless of their illness; this can be accommodated by changing the times of oral medications or replacing them with formulations that can be administered via another route (eg, intravenous, intranasal, transdermal, rectal), at least during daylight hours. Diagnostic studies, such as barium swallows, should be scheduled for after sunset, if possible, at which time a Muslim has broken his or her fast and can eat and drink by mouth. Fasting diabetic patients continue to require insulin. With the help of an endocrinologist, it may be possible for diabetic Muslim patients to receive intravenous insulin injections or long-acting oral medication.

Older Muslims with a weak constitution, or any Muslim adult who is ill from an acute, chronic, or incurable disease, are exempt from fasting.

Barriers to Quality Health Care Among Muslims

Language

Language is often a barrier to adequate health care among older immigrant Muslims. Over 90% of the world's Muslims live in countries where English is not the primary or commonly spoken language. The most frequently spoken languages in the Muslim world are Malay, Urdu, Hausa, Arabic, and Farsi/Dari. Delayed acculturation and language barriers tend to restrict older patients' access to adequate health information and preventive screening programs. Translated information and mosque-based screening programs can provide effective outreach for older non-English speaking patients. A competent, hospital-certified interpreter, of whom the patient approves, is very helpful.

Culture and Religion

Illness has many meanings in Islam and Muslim cultures. Many Muslims show a high level of acceptance of their illness, because they view it as a purification of their sins. Others may express great fear if they perceive their illness as Divine wrath or punishment, or due to the "evil eye" from jealous people. Some patients may reject allopathic treatments, because they see the etiology of their illness as spiritual or metaphysical in nature. Acknowledging a patient's perceived metaphysical concerns, rather than dismissing them, while pointing out the possibilities in treatment of the physical symptoms can reconcile the differing views between the medical team and the patient and can facilitate patient acceptance of medical treatments as a "supplement" to spiritual cures.

> *Many Muslims show a high level of acceptance of their illness, because they view it as a purification of their sins.*

Family plays an important role in the healing process and support for the sick and elderly among Muslims. This could translate into a larger number of visitors and self-designated surrogate decision makers for a patient. Facilitating Islamic acts of worship is paramount for religious, older Muslim patients to feel well cared for in the hospital.

Roles for Spiritual Leaders or Advisors in Health Care Settings

Older Muslims and their families may rely on a religious scholar or leader—referred to as "Imam," "Sheikh," or "Mullah"—to provide spiritual support, explain theological principles, perform rituals, offer prayers, or answer questions regarding the religious ruling on certain medical treatments, procedures, or options such as organ donation and withdrawal of life support. Many hospital chaplaincies keep contact information for nearby mosques and Muslim scholars who can be reached for support of Muslim patients and their families. In grave situations, the role of the religious scholar, who uses language that is derived from the Islamic worldview, can be crucial in supporting older Muslims and their families.

Disclosure and Consent

Islam places a high degree of importance on autonomy. If a family member requests that information about health status or risks of procedures not be given to a patient, the consensual and voluntary nature of this decision should be ascertained. Often, family members are concerned about the emotional impact of bad news and wish to shield the patient for this reason, not in an effort to deny patient autonomy. Therefore, family members may not be best suited for the role of interpreter for serious medical discussions. A recent study suggests that older Muslims wish to receive frank and full disclosure more than had been thought previously.

> *A recent study suggests that older Muslims wish to receive frank and full disclosure more than had been thought previously.*

Views on Do-Not-Resuscitate Orders, Nutrition, and Hydration at End of Life

Islam emphasizes the sanctity of life over the quality of life. If a person is suffering from an acute illness or an acute flare-up of a chronic illness and has a chance of surviving, then all reasonable interventions should be considered. Hastening death by any means is forbidden. These include suicide, passive euthanasia (in which an intervention is withheld for an illness that could be cured or mitigated), or active euthanasia (in which a beneficial intervention is withdrawn, or an intervention is performed that knowingly results in death). However, if the disease is so advanced that intervention is only delaying death, or the treatment of a terminal illness causes more suffering than the illness itself, then a do-not-resuscitate order is acceptable. The health care team's ability to recognize medical futility and to convey it, compassionately and gradually, to a Muslim family can be a great aid in allowing for palliative care and preparing the family for end-of-life rituals.

> *Hastening death by any means is forbidden.*

Nutrition and hydration are considered basic human needs in Islam and therefore are not considered to be extraordinary care. Ceasing nutritional support is considered a form of passive euthanasia.

Advance Directives

Advance directives are not common among Muslims. Advance directives that allow for passive or active euthanasia or assisted suicide are not permissible. However, an advance directive that delineates criteria for do-not-resuscitate orders (by the conditions mentioned previously), palliative care, final rights, and burial preparations is ideal and should be encouraged. Ideally, a care facility and a local Muslim center would work together to develop advance directives that could be made available to Muslim patients, preferably in the languages commonly spoken among Muslim patients in the area.

Views on Palliative Care

Seeking treatment is recommended but is not obligatory for incurable diseases. The decision to discontinue futile interventions and transition to palliative care is a hard one for many older Muslims and their families, given the patient's position within the family. The rationale behind the recommendation for such a decision needs to be explained to the patient and his or her family using culturally and religiously sensitive language. For example, it is not appropriate to place a term on the life expectancy of the patient, unless the patient/family asks. At this stage, the family may adamantly desire to conceal from the patient the status of his or her medical condition. The patient's informed consent to such desire should be ascertained.

Seeking treatment is recommended but is not obligatory for incurable diseases.

The use of pain medication, including sedatives and opioids, to alleviate suffering is permissible when medically necessary. It is strongly recommended that the patient be informed of the available options regarding pain medication, including times of administration and effects, so that he or she has a chance to arrange timed religious duties, such as prayer.

When hospice or home care is needed, the health care team should seek clarification from the older Muslim and his or her family on religious and personal preferences that would make the patient comfortable. For example, while hospitalized and especially at time of death, some Muslims are not comfortable being surrounded by any statues or drawings, especially non-Islamic religious art. They may request same-sex health care providers. Patients can be expected to need visitations by a religious leader. Large numbers of visitors from family, friends, and fellow community members is expected.

Death is considered a passing stage between this life and the life to come.

Beliefs About Death and Life After Death

Death is considered a passing stage between this life and the life to come. It is the departure of the spirit from the body. Around the time of death, all family members, sometimes including children, want to be present to reaffirm the cardinal beliefs of the Islamic faith with the patient.

Once the patient has died, most Muslim families proceed immediately with funeral arrangements. Paperwork should be completed expeditiously. Same-sex health care providers are preferred to handle the body after death.

| CASE STUDY **1** | **Health Care Procedures and Cultural Needs for Modesty** |

Objectives

1. Consider the role of communication and the role of family when an older Muslim patient is hospitalized.
2. Describe the impact of language and cultural barriers to optimal health care.
3. Discuss the need for advance directives and do-not-resuscitate orders.
4. List some important end-of-life rituals.
5. Discuss the impact of health care workers' own culture on transcultural understanding.

Mrs. Khan, a 72-year-old, non-English speaking Indian Muslim, has severe coronary artery disease. Despite being a high-risk candidate, she undergoes balloon angioplasty on the advice of her son, who is a physician. Shortly after the procedure, Mrs. Khan develops complications. Her son alerts the nurse and asks that something be done. The nurse pages the resident and waits for a callback. The son notes that Mrs. Khan's health status is continuing to deteriorate and becomes agitated and insists that a physician be notified again. The nurse places Mrs. Khan on oxygen and leaves. The son continues to insist a physician be called, and he is forcibly removed from the intensive care unit by security.

Question:

1. How could the nurse have approached the situation with Mrs. Khan's son differently?

The nurse could have attempted to understand the source of Dr. Khan's emotional distress, paged a resident or attending physician on the public address system to speak with Dr. Khan, or contacted her nursing supervisor to speak with Dr. Khan.

Mrs. Khan's condition further deteriorated and an electrocardiogram was obtained, necessitating that her chest be partially exposed.

Question:

1. How could Mrs. Khan's Islamic belief in modesty have been accommodated when it was necessary to expose her chest for the electrocardiogram?

After the leads for the electrocardiogram had been placed, Mrs. Khan's gown could have been drawn up over her chest.

Mrs. Khan later experienced an unstable heart rhythm, and a "code blue" was called. A number of resident physicians, mostly men, rushed in, completely exposing Mrs. Khan's chest. Chest compressions were performed, unsuccessfully, and Mrs. Khan died a few minutes later. The son later remarked, "I failed my mother. She died cold, alone, and half-naked. This is how I will always remember my mother's death."

Question:

1. While it was appropriate for male residents to perform the resuscitation on Mrs. Khan as a life-saving procedure, what could have been said to the family afterward to allay their concern of the violation of gender preferences?

The health care team could have explained that because of the emergent situation, every attempt was made to save her life and that under other circumstances, every effort would have been made to accommodate Mrs. Khan's sense of modesty.

Question:

1. How could accommodations have been made for end-of-life rituals when it was clear that Mrs. Khan's clinical status was deteriorating?

A family member, such as Mrs. Khan's son, could have been allowed back in, or a chaplain notified.

Question:

1. Would an advance directive have been helpful in clarifying the wishes of the family?

Despite the fact that Mrs. Khan's son was a physician, and despite the cardiologist's reservation in doing the procedure, the family did not clearly express to the health care team Mrs. Khan's or the family's wishes in the event of serious morbidity or even death. These preferences are difficult to establish when a patient is close to death. An advance directive could be very helpful before an invasive procedure in a high-risk patient. The cardiologist could have asked for a palliative care consult or discussed the risks and benefits of the procedure directly with the patient, using language interpretation services.

CASE STUDY 2 | The Diversity of Muslim Patients

Objectives

1. Appreciate the impact of universal human needs, such as the need to feel well cared for, on the behavior of any patient regardless of ethnicity or spiritual belief.
2. Understand ways by which the medical team can deal with the differing experiences of Muslim patients and their families.
3. Highlight the importance of opening communication channels between the patient and the medical team to determine the patient's needs.
4. Identify and seek the help of Muslim staff within the health care facility who can assist the medical team in understanding concerns of Muslim patients.

Mr. Aref Farhadi is a 75-year-old Iranian American Muslim who immigrated to the United States with his wife and adult children when he was 65. He speaks English competently, albeit with a heavy accent. Mr. and Mrs. Farhadi live with their oldest son and daughter-in-law. Mr. Farhadi has a history of diabetes. He started complaining of chest and leg pain, for which his doctor prescribed a short hospitalization for diagnostic tests and to make sure the diabetes was well controlled.

Mrs. Farhadi was continually at her husband's bedside, and their children took turns visiting both of them. The first day went well for Mr. Farhadi, and he complied fully with his treatment regimen. On his second day of hospitalization, however, the bedside nurse reported that Mr. Farhadi adamantly refused to take his morning insulin injection. The medical team was puzzled because all the health care providers, including a hospital Muslim volunteer who visited earlier, had indicated having a pleasant and smooth interaction with Mr. Farhadi and his family.

Question:

1. How do you think the medical team should approach the situation with Mr. Farhadi?

The medical team could identify one of the health care providers who had previously interacted with the family and have this provider ask Mr. Farhadi and his family why he was now refusing to take his insulin. Whenever possible, health care providers are also advised to seek the counsel of chaplaincy staff. A chaplaincy intervention becomes crucial when members of the medical team find themselves passing moral judgments on the decisions, wishes, or behaviors of patients or their families who are from a different ethnic or religious background.

The medical team tried to put together some theories why Mr. Farhadi was refusing insulin and unanimously concluded that he was probably trying to avoid receiving porcine insulin. Earlier, two of his health care providers indicated that Mr. Farhadi is a devout Muslim because he was keen on performing the Islamic prayer while in bed. The team agreed to make a referral to chaplaincy to have the Muslim volunteer address the issue further with Mr. Farhadi.

Arriving at the patient's room, Ahsan Ali—the Muslim volunteer—found that Mr. Farhadi was asleep. Mrs. Farhadi was there with her two sons, and she welcomed Mr. Ali into the room. Dinner had just arrived, and Mr. Ali immediately noted that Mr. Farhadi's older son was meticulously checking his father's dinner, reading all labels, and ensuring a diabetic diet. Seeing Mr. Ali's puzzled look at his behavior, the son casually added, "You know they brought my father a regular person's diet this morning. He almost went into shock. I am trying to make sure he gets the right diet now!"

Question:
1. Now, why do you think Mr. Farhadi was refusing his insulin?

Although it was perfectly reasonable to assume that Mr. Farhadi was trying to avoid receiving porcine insulin, especially given his devoutness, the health care providers could have benefited from keeping other possible options open for why the patient was refusing the medical treatment. A crucial element of cultural competency is the ability to discern whether the patient's culture is the major drive for his or her behavior. In this case, Mr. Farhadi had lost trust in the health care providers after he received the wrong breakfast, and he reacted by refusing to take his insulin. Mr. Farhadi was aware that he was receiving porcine insulin and did not object in principle because he understood it was a life-saving medication.

Kamyar M. Hedayat, MD
Doha R. Hamza
Ahmed Nezar M. Kobeisy, PhD

References

American Muslims: Population statistics. Available at: http://www.cair-net.org/asp/populationstats.asp (accessed April 2007).

Bader A, Musshauser D, Sahin F, Bezirkan H, Hochleitner M. The Mosque campaign: a cardiovascular prevention program for female Turkish immigrants. *Wien Klin Wochenschr* 2006;118(7–8):217–223.

Ebrahim AF. The living will (Wasiyat Al-Hayy): a study of its legality in the light of Islamic jurisprudence. *Med Law* 2000;19(1):147–160.

Haniff GM. The Muslim community in America: a brief profile. *J Muslim Minority Affairs* 2003;23(2):303–311.

Hedayat KM, Pirzadeh R. Issues in Islamic biomedical ethics: a primer for the pediatrician. *Pediatrics* 2001;108(4):965–971.

Hedayat KM. When the spirit leaves: childhood death, grieving and bereavement in Islam. *J Palliat Care* 2006;9(6):1286–1291.

Lipson JG, Omidian PA. Health issues of Afghan refugees in California. *West J Med* 1992;157(3):271–275.

Luna L. Care and cultural context of Lebanese Muslim immigrants: using Leininger's theory. *J Transcult Nurs* 1994;5(2):12–20.

Morioka-Douglas N, Sacks T, Yeo G. Issues in caring for Afghan American elders: insights from literature and a focus group. *J Cross Cult Gerontol* 2004;19(1):27–40.

Omeri A. Culture care of Iranian immigrants in New South Wales, Australia: sharing transcultural nursing knowledge. *J Transcult Nurs* 1997;8(2):5–16.

Rulings on physical examination and diagnosis. In: Rohani M, Noghani F (eds). *Ahkam-e Pezeshi*. Tehran, Iran: Teymurzadeh Cultural Publication Foundation; 1998.

Additional Resources

1. The Islamic Society of North America. Available at: www.isna.net (accessed April 2007). An umbrella group and the largest Muslim organization in North America; has extensive resources and links to resources within the Muslim community.

2. Imamia Medics International. Available at: http://imamiamedics.org/ (accessed April 2007). International Shia Medical Humanitarian organization; Web site contains articles on Islamic ethics including organ transplantation, bereavement and grieving, and other topics. IMI has an extensive list of physicians and clerics available for consultation.

3. The Islamic Medical Association of North America. Available at: www.imana.org/mc/page.do (accessed April 2007). IMANA published a brochure on Islamic medical ethics that is available on its Web site.

4. The Muslim Spiritual Care Service at Stanford Hospital. Available at: www.stanfordhospital.com/forPatients/patientServices/chaplaincyServices (accessed April 2007). This group offers cultural competency training on care of Islam and Muslim patients, in addition to providing resources, brochures, and other documents on the care of Muslim patients and their families.

5. Hold Your Breath: a Journey into Cross-cultural Medicine. Available at: http://medethicsfilms.stanford.edu/holdyourbreath/ (accessed April 2007). A documentary film highlighting the plight of Muhammad Kochi, an older Afghan Muslim patient, and the interaction between traditional Western medical culture and traditional Muslim belief.

6. Islamic Networks Group. Available at: www.ing.org (accessed April 2007). A nonprofit organization that offers presentations on Islam and Muslim cultures in various disciplines including health care.

CHAPTER 7

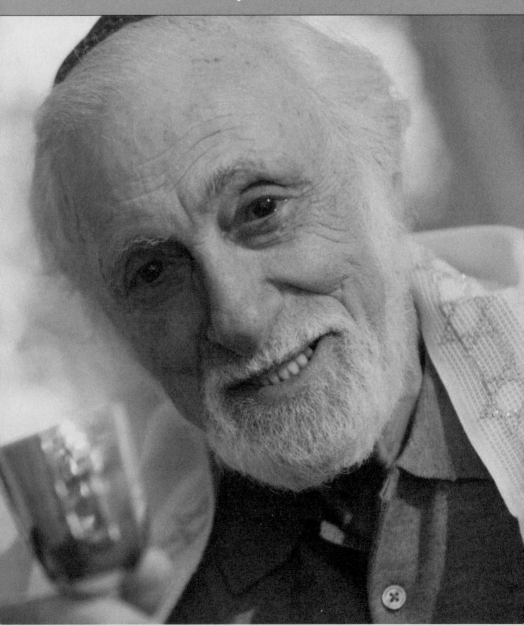

Judaism

Knowledge and observance of Jewish customs and religious practice vary widely among Jews. Traditional beliefs and practices may or may not be relevant for given individuals and their families, particularly those who have little knowledge of Judaism but strongly identify themselves as being Jewish in a cultural way. When taking a clinical history, it is useful to include a question such as, "So I can best take care of you, do you have any spiritual or religious observances or beliefs that are meaningful to you, that you would like me to be aware of?"

History

Judaism, which gave rise to Christianity and Islam, is the religion of nearly 14 million Jews worldwide. Jews identify themselves by religion, culture, and/or history. The largest concentration of Jews live in Israel and the United States. According to Jewish tradition, Jewish history began nearly 4000 years ago in the land that is Israel, founded by Abraham approximately 1850 BCE. Judaism affirms the oneness of God and that human beings are made in the image of God, that human beings are given freedom of choice, and that they serve as God's partner in completing creation. There are also Jews who don't believe in God, but who embrace Judaism as a system of ethics, culture, and history.

> *According to Jewish tradition, Jewish history began nearly 4000 years ago in the land that is Israel, founded by Abraham approximately 1850 BCE.*

Judaism stresses performance of commandments, *mitzvot,* rather than adherence to a belief system. Central authority in Judaism is not vested in any person or group but rather in Judaism's sacred writings, laws, and traditions. These sacred writings begin with Moses, who led the Israelites from Egyptian captivity and back to Israel approximately 1280 BCE. After the second temple in Jerusalem was destroyed by the Romans in 70 CE, Jews migrated to central Asia, North Africa, the Mediterranean, and Europe. Antisemitism, leading to multiple expulsions and destruction of Jewish communities, has resulted in Jews living at one time or another in almost every country of the world.

During the Middle Ages, significant differences in language, liturgy, and culture developed between the Sephardic Jews, centered in Spain, and the Ashkenazic Jews, centered in France and Germany. In 19th-century Europe after the Enlightenment, Reform and Conservative denominations of Judaism developed in contrast to Orthodoxy. European Judaism suffered terribly from 1933 to 1945 during the Holocaust, when six million Jews were put to death by the Nazis. In 1948, the modern state of Israel was founded.

The first Jews in America emigrated from Holland in the 1600s, fleeing the Spanish and Portuguese Inquisitions.

The first Jews in America emigrated from Holland in the 1600s, fleeing the Spanish and Portuguese Inquisitions. The next major wave of Jewish immigrants arrived in the 1800s–1920s, escaping devastating massacres of entire villages (pogroms) in Russia and eastern Europe. Those escaping the Nazis came in the 1930s, and those who survived the *Shoah*, the Holocaust, in the 1950s. Since the 1980s, many Jews have emigrated from the former Soviet Union, North Africa, and the Middle East, including Israel.

American Jewish communities have created strong communal infrastructures since they first arrived in the United States. Jewish communal groups typically include synagogues, Jewish Federations (which help other Jewish organizations locally and in Israel), Jewish Community Centers (a gathering place with recreational, social, and religious programming), Jewish Homes for the Aged, Jewish Family and Children's Services (providing social services for all ages including older adults), Jewish funeral homes and burial societies, and Hebrew Free Loan Associations (providing emergency financial assistance with no interest). Some communities now include a Jewish Healing Center (providing spiritual care for Jews living with illness, loss, and other significant life challenges).

Daily life is made holy by the emphasis on the ritual fitness of foods, the recitation of blessings for a variety of everyday acts, and prayer services.

Important Holidays and Celebrations

Judaism has a rich and textured cycle of yearly holidays, prescribed daily activities, and life-cycle events. Daily life is made holy by the emphasis on the ritual fitness of foods, the recitation of blessings for a variety of everyday acts, and prayer services.

The Jewish calendar is based on a combination of the lunar and solar (Gregorian) calendars. The day begins and ends at sunset, and the month begins with the new moon. The year is 12 lunar months long and lags behind the solar calendar by 11 days. An extra month is added every 2–3 years to synchronize with the solar calendar. Thus, the dates of Jewish holidays vary from year to year on the Gregorian calendar. When a Jewish holiday is listed on the Gregorian calendar, it begins at sundown the day before.

The weekly Sabbath—from sundown Friday to sundown Saturday—is considered the most important religious holiday. It is based on the Bible: "On the seventh day, God rested." Observant Jews who closely follow Sabbath religious observance refrain from working, driving, writing, and using electricity. In health care settings, this can affect traveling, using elevators, signing papers, preparing for funerals, and removing the body after death. Observant Jews may need assistance in observing Sabbath and dietary laws during hospitalization or while living in a long-term-care facility. A Jewish hospital chaplain or rabbi can be of assistance.

> *The weekly Sabbath—from sundown Friday to sundown Saturday—is considered the most important religious holiday.*

The yearly cycle of religious holidays begins in early to mid-fall with the high holidays of *Rosh Hashanah* (the Jewish New Year) and *Yom Kippur* (the holiest day, a fast day of atonement). These are immediately followed by *Sukkot* (the harvest festival of booths). *Hanukah* (the festival of lights) is in December, followed by *Purim* in late winter. Passover (the most-celebrated Jewish holiday, commemorating the exodus from Egypt) is in early spring, and *Shavuot* (the celebration of receiving the Ten Commandments) in late spring.

Each holiday has particular rituals and foods that have symbolic value. For example, Jews will fast on *Yom Kippur*. On the 8 nights of *Hanukah*, they light candles in a *menorah*, a special candelabra. During the 8 days of Passover, *matzah* (unleavened bread that the Jews ate during the exodus from Egypt) is eaten, and foods made of leavened grains are avoided. Jews of different cultural traditions celebrate holidays in different ways with foods, clothing, melodies, and design of ritual items that reflect the cultural and aesthetic influence of their countries of origin.

> *Each holiday has particular rituals and foods that have symbolic value.*

Life-cycle events include circumcising boys on day 8 after birth, naming girls in synagogues, and celebrating the religious adulthood of boys and girls *(bar/bat mitzvah)* at age 13, marriages, and funerals. Many families make great efforts, including traveling long distances, to gather for holidays and life-cycle events. Traditionally, Jews have placed great emphasis on marriage within Judaism, strongly discouraging interfaith marriages, such as those between Jews and Christians. However, given the high rate of interfaith marriages, liberal streams of Judaism are more accepting of such unions when children are raised Jewish.

Sacred Objects and Scriptures

The *Torah* scroll (a parchment written in ancient Hebrew) contains the first five books of the Hebrew Bible *(Tanakh)*. It is so sacred that Jews have often entered burning synagogues to retrieve the *Torah* scrolls. Other sacred items include prayer books and the *mezuzah* (an inscribed parchment inside a case hung on entryways to buildings). Candles are lit to mark the beginning of *Shabbat* and holidays, on the 8 nights of *Hanukah*, for the 7 days after a burial, and on the anniversary of a death.

Jews may wear religious garments. Observant men (and now some women as well) may wear an undergarment with knotted tassels on each corner *(tallit katan)*, a skullcap *(yarmulke* or *kippah)*, leather boxes containing prayers that are strapped onto the forehead and upper arm during prayer *(tefillin* or phylacteries), and a large prayer shawl *(tallit)*.

> *Observant Jewish women follow strict customs relating to modesty (*tzniut *or* tznius*), wearing a wig or scarf to cover the hair, and long dresses and long sleeves to cover the body.*

Observant Jewish women follow strict customs relating to modesty *(tzniut* or *tznius)*, wearing a wig or scarf to cover the hair, and long dresses and long sleeves to cover the body. Removing one's clothing and wearing hospital gowns can challenge this sensibility.

Both observant and nonobservant Jews may wear jewelry with Jewish symbols. Some are worn for their perceived protective value (to ward off bad luck or bring good health), while others are worn as an expression of religious commitment and/or pride of cultural identity.

The twin pillars of Judaism are the Hebrew Bible *(Tanakh)* and the *Talmud*. The *Torah*, the first five books of the Hebrew Bible, chronicles the early history of the Jews and is the ultimate source of the law on which Jews rely for moral guidance. The term Old Testament is often considered pejorative, because it can be interpreted as being inferior or outdated relative to the New Testament. In addition to the Hebrew Bible, a vast sacred literature has developed over the past two millennia, including the *Talmud* (a collection of commentaries on the Bible) and books of prayer. New sacred texts continue to be written to this day. From these writings emerge the laws and stories that embody the central Jewish values of life, family, education, community, social justice, memory, continuity across the generations, and *tikun olam* (repair of the world).

Diverse Subgroups

In the United States, 2.1% of the population (6.4 million people) are Jewish, the majority having immigrated from Europe. Nearly 8% of all American Jews immigrated to the United States since 1980. Approximately two-thirds came from the former Soviet Union and the rest from Israel, Canada, Iran, South Africa, and over 25 other countries. Most American Jews are highly educated, but there are also many impoverished and working class Jews. One in five Jews is 65 or older (20%), nearly double the national average (12.4%). Of older Jewish adults, one-third live alone, 67% are widows or widowers, and 9% live below the federally defined poverty line.

In the United States, 2.1% of the population (6.4 million people) are Jewish, the majority having immigrated from Europe.

Religious observance and involvement in tradition and community vary widely. Three-fourths of American Jews identify by religious denomination (Orthodox 10%, Conservative 27%, Reform 35%, Reconstructionist 2%, Renewal <1%, and Humanist <1%) and the rest as "just Jewish" (25%). Approximately one-third are members of synagogues.

Many older immigrant Jews who fled oppression and persecution may purposefully hide their religious preference in the hospital. Because the former Soviet Union threatened imprisonment or death for practicing Judaism, many Jewish immigrants/refugees from that area identify strongly as being Jewish but have little or no religious or historical knowledge of their heritage.

Many older immigrant Jews who fled oppression and persecution may purposefully hide their religious preference in the hospital.

Roles of Spiritual Leaders and Advisors in Health Care Issues

Jews who belong to a synagogue may turn to their rabbi, cantor, or congregation's lay members for pastoral care. In the community outside the synagogue, they may call on rabbis, chaplains, psychologists, social workers, or spiritual directors who may be affiliated with the local Jewish Federation, Jewish Family and Children's Service, Jewish Home for the Aged, or a local hospital. Jewish pastoral support involves listening, providing guidance, and offering prayer. It can also include referrals for communal resources such as food, transportation, housing, or counseling. Some families, particularly those who are Orthodox, will consult with a rabbi for medical decisions. In these situations, decisions are made in conjunction with the health care providers, the patient (or family or surrogate), and the rabbi.

Religious Basis for Views of Health and Disease

Jewish life is infused with sacred religious obligations called *mitzvot*. Examples include keeping the Sabbath, fasting on *Yom Kippur*, observing the kosher dietary laws, honoring one's parents, and visiting the sick. Because human beings are formed in the image of the Divine, life is regarded as sacred and considered of infinite value regardless of its duration or quality. Preserving life is regarded as a cardinal value. This value, called *pikuach nefesh*, supersedes almost all the commandments of the *Torah*. Even on *Yom Kippur*, the holiest day of the year when fasting is obligated, those who are sick, pregnant, or nursing are obligated to eat.

Taking care of one's body is a *mitzvah*. One's body is not one's own, but rather a gift from God. Human beings are the caretakers of this sacred gift. Autopsy is discouraged out of concern for violating the sanctity of the body, except when the information would serve to save a life or when legally required. Nevertheless, *pikuach nefesh* is so important that all Jews are encouraged to donate bodily organs so that others may live.

Taking care of one's body is a mitzvah. *One's body is not one's own, but rather a gift from God.*

In Jewish theology, the body and soul are integrated. In the morning prayers, a Jew thanks God for organs that work and gives thanks for the stages of awakening, such as opening one's eyes and then standing up. Jewish tradition enthusiastically supports the practice of medicine, in which healing is seen as a partnership with God. From ancient times to the present, Judaism has understood that health is affected by the availability

Jewish tradition enthusiastically supports the practice of medicine, in which healing is seen as a partnership with God.

and use of medical techniques, as well as by prayer and spiritual support. Thus, healing involves prayer, religious observance, and the work of a physician. In fact, Jewish teaching asserts that one should live in a town where there is a physician. Preventive medicine and self-care is detailed in the Bible and in the 12th-century writings of Moses Maimonides, the Jewish physician, philosopher, and rabbinic scholar.

Understanding illness reflects one's theology and relationship to the Divine. For some, illness is simply a natural manifestation of life, while for others, illness may be experienced as a punishment.

Visiting the sick, *bikur cholim*, is a very important *mitzvah* and is provided by family, friends, and members of the community. Jewish tradition provides guidelines on visiting the sick, eg, sitting at or below the level of the patient's head. It is said that visiting the sick removes one-sixtieth of the sick person's illness, suggesting that the caring presence of loved ones and members of the community can make an appreciable difference in the person's experience of illness and suffering. It is a *mitzvah* to visit both Jews and non-Jews.

Dietary Restrictions

Kashrut is the body of Jewish law dealing with what foods Jews can and cannot eat, and how those foods must be prepared and eaten. The term "kosher" describes foods and ritual objects that are made in accordance with Jewish law.

Milk products and meat products may not be cooked or eaten together. It is permissible to eat fish with fins and scales, and meat from cows, sheep, and poultry. Shellfish and pork are not permissible. Meat products from permissible animals is kosher only if the animal is ritually slaughtered in a way that minimizes pain and is inspected to be free of disease. Items that are labeled kosher or carry a kosher icon signify rabbinic supervision of the preparation of the food.

Items that are labeled kosher or carry a kosher icon signify rabbinic supervision of the preparation of the food.

Gender Considerations

The role of women varies widely among denominations. In traditional Orthodox Judaism, the roles of men and women are clearly demarcated. For instance, worship services are always led by men, and women and men sit separately. Women practice rituals that men do not, such as lighting Sabbath candles. In Orthodox communities that follow the customs of modesty *(tzniut* or *tznius)*, men and women who are not married or closely related are not allowed to shake hands, touch each other, or be alone in a private room.

In the United States, since the 1920s, feminism has been growing among Jewish women. Now, thousands of egalitarian communities exist throughout the country, where women participate in the same religious rituals and customs as men. Many older women who were previously excluded from participating in Jewish ritual leadership are now leading their communities in worship and life-cycle events and having adult *bat mitzvah.* For many older immigrant women, learning these skills is especially poignant, because it creates a profound contrast between the lives they led as young girls and the lives they now have in their new country.

Healing and Health-Promoting Ceremonies and Rituals

Judaism encompasses myriad health-promoting ceremonies and rituals.

Judaism encompasses myriad health-promoting ceremonies and rituals. The important *mitzvah* of *bikur cholim,* visiting the sick, has already been discussed. Individual and communal daily prayers include prayers for healing. They may be recited by an individual for oneself, or by others on one's behalf. On days when the *Torah* is read, a special prayer, the *misheberach,* is read for all who are ill or suffering. This is recited using the person's Hebrew name (traditionally) or English name. It can be deeply moving to be asked one's name for a *misheberach,* at times bringing tears even to those who do not consider themselves to be religious. For centuries, some 30 psalms, including Psalms 6, 9, 13, 23, 31, and 103, have been recognized as especially effective for bringing hope and solace to those who are suffering.

Names are recognized as having great power. When a person is very ill, there is a custom to alter their Hebrew name by adding a new one. A typical new first name would include the Hebrew word for life, for blessing, or for the name of someone who has lived many years.

More recently, Jewish communities have begun holding special healing services that may involve singing, reciting prayers and psalms, and group sharing. This recent phenomenon in the American Jewish society may be unfamiliar to older Jews, especially recent immigrants.

Beliefs about Death and Life After Death

Judaism emphasizes that a person is fully a person until the very last breath, and that life is sacred, no matter the quality. However, this does not imply that life should be prolonged at all costs. Although *pikuach nefesh*, saving a life, is an extremely high value, Judaism nonetheless respects that death is inevitable. Jews should neither hasten death nor prolong the dying process. Judaism does not support suicide or assisted suicide.

Jews should neither hasten death nor prolong the dying process.

Beliefs regarding the afterlife vary widely among Jews from "nothing exists beyond this life on earth" to "there is a definite existence for the soul after life." In both cases, Jews believe one lives on through being remembered by others. There are also beliefs in bodily resurrection of the dead and, for some, in reincarnation. Rarely does the dying Jewish person or family find comfort in focusing on the afterlife. Greater comfort accrues from having left a good name and in knowing that one will be remembered honorably. Memory and legacy are essential values in Judaism.

Rarely does the dying Jewish person or family find comfort in focusing on the afterlife.

Views on Do-Not-Resuscitate Orders, Nutrition, and Hydration at End of Life

Jewish belief that life is sacred and of infinite value does not necessarily translate into maintaining life at all costs. When death is inevitable, Judaism allows for the withdrawal of life-support technologies and the removal of obstacles to dying. Opinions vary widely on these topics. For individual patients, one should inquire about their particular beliefs, and consult with a Jewish chaplain or rabbi as needed.

When death is inevitable, Judaism allows for the withdrawal of life-support technologies and the removal of obstacles to dying.

If a patient is dying of a terminal disease, some would say that any life must be preserved under all circumstances. Many others would relinquish aggressive medical treatment, even if it is effective in maintaining vital organs. In grave situations, Judaism allows for steps to be taken to relieve pain or other symptoms even if such actions could inadvertently hasten death, as long as the intent is clearly on treating pain or symptoms and not on terminating life. A patient may undergo a life-threatening procedure that offers only a slight hope of cure, but he or she is not obligated to do so.

In terminal or incurable illness, life-sustaining treatments such as chemotherapy or antibiotics may be discontinued, and do-not-resuscitate or do-not-intubate orders may be issued. This is not considered terminating a life. Within Judaism, opinions differ regarding nutrition and hydration. When these are delivered through a feeding tube or intravenous line, some authorities consider them medicine that may be withheld; others consider them as basic sustenance that must be provided.

Hospice use among Jewish families is demonstrably low.

With regard to hospice and palliative care, hospice use among Jewish families is demonstrably low. Many Jews may resist because of Judaism's emphasis on the value of life and because of having a "survivor mentality," thinking that to be Jewish means to fight death at all costs. This is changing with the increasing involvement of rabbis and Jewish chaplains in community and Jewish hospices.

The experience during the Holocaust may be a factor in medical care for survivors of the concentration camps, their children, and extended family. Some areas of increased sensitivity include bathing or showering, medical testing, nutritional status and weight loss, perception of pain and suffering, views of death itself, importance of memory, multiple losses, and grief.

Religious Customs and Rituals for Dying Patients and After Death

Performing a life review with the dying person is in keeping with the focus of this life on earth, good deeds, and the legacy of the deceased. An ethical will can be prepared by the dying person (or at any stage of life). It allows one to share with others, in his or her own words, some of life's lessons, memories, hopes and dreams, beliefs and values.

Before dying, certain prayers are recited. Most common are the *Shema*, the central statement of faith *(Shema Yisrael, Adonai Eloheinu, Adonai Echad*–Hear O Israel, the Lord is our God, the Lord is One); the *Vidui*, a confessional prayer; and Psalms. These are recited by the individual, if possible, or by a Jewish clergy or chaplain. It is just as acceptable, and sometimes more meaningful, for these prayers to be recited by a family member or a close friend. They may be recited even after the person has lost consciousness.

After death, Judaism prescribes practices for preparing the body, burial, and mourning. These are of great significance, including for many who are not otherwise religious in belief or observance. From the time of death until the funeral, the body should be attended by a *shomer* (guard) to honor the person by not leaving the body alone. The family may fulfill this duty or assign someone to do so.

After death, Judaism prescribes practices for preparing the body, burial, and mourning.

Judaism emphasizes that all are equal in death. Traditionally, Jews are shrouded in linen clothes and buried in plain wooden boxes without any metal. Traditional preparation for burial, *Tahar* (washing the body and reciting prayers), is done by volunteers of the holy burial society *(Chevre Kaddisha)* in keeping with religious laws that preserve respect for the dead. The funeral and burial usually take place as soon as possible, typically within 24–72 hours but not on the Sabbath or holy days.

Cremation is not supported by Jewish law, particularly in light of the Holocaust. Cremation can be a source of conflict and debate within a family, even for nonreligious Jews. Nonetheless, an increasing number of Jews elect cremation (25%–30%), and the ashes are either buried or scattered.

Cremation is not supported by Jewish law, particularly in light of the Holocaust.

After burial, Judaism prescribes periods of time for mourning one's immediate family. This includes a 3- to7-day period called *shiva* for staying at home and being visited by the community, and a 30-day period called *shloshim* for returning to work but refraining from entertainment. The period of mourning for the death of spouses, siblings, and children is 30 days; for parents it is 1 year. During the period of mourning, a special mourner's prayer is said daily. A monument is unveiled during the first year. A special 24-hour memorial candle is lit on the anniversary of the death, the *yahrzeit,* and four times a year during the holidays of *Yom Kippur, Sukkot,* Passover, and *Shavuot.*

| CASE STUDY **1** | **Community and Social Roles of Religious Organizations** |

Objective

1. Identify resources in the Jewish community for supporting older adults and their families.

Dr. Maureen Kelly's next two patients are scheduled together for an extended visit. They are Sarah Roth, an 84-year-old Caucasian woman and her 88-year-old husband, Irving. The Roths are American Jews born of Russian immigrant parents. They are fond of Dr. Kelly, whom they've known for a long time. The Roth's married daughter, Rachel, has two teenage sons and lives out of town. She keeps in touch daily by telephone and visits every 2 months. Today, Rachel brings her parents to discuss some changes in their situation. Mrs. Roth has started to wander at night and is sleeping more during the day. She needs help showering and sometimes with toileting. Mrs. Roth's clothes seem to have more food stains than in the past. Mr. Roth says he can't clean the clothes well because his cataracts and glaucoma are getting worse. Rachel thinks her father cannot care for her mother by himself, because her mother needs more social stimulation and medical supervision than he can provide.

Mrs. Roth is a retired homemaker with early-stage dementia, hypothyroidism, and high cholesterol. Her medications are donepezil, atorvastatin, and thyroid replacement therapy. Mr. Roth, a retired tailor, has been taking care of shopping, meals, driving, laundry, and medications. Recently, he began helping his wife with bathing and toileting, which has been embarrassing for them both. A housekeeper comes in weekly to help with the cleaning. Mr. Roth has mild hypertension and glaucoma and takes hydrochlorothiazide and eye drops. He is a meticulous man who takes pride in caring for his wife and himself. Their modest income comes from savings, social security, and a reverse mortgage.

Dr. Kelly compliments Mr. Roth on his dedication in taking care of Mrs. Roth. Referring to the biblical phrase "For everything there is a season, a time for everything under heaven," she suggests that this might be the time for Mr. Roth to get some help at home and to get some respite through daytime activities for Mrs. Roth. Mr. Roth agrees that his wife would benefit from increased stimulation. He reluctantly agrees to more assistance at home but does not know how to accomplish this.

Question:

1. What are some resources in the Jewish community that are available for older adults?

Dr. Kelly suggests that social and religious organizations can be of help. Mr. Roth says, "We're not what you would call religious people. We don't keep kosher and go to synagogue only on the high holidays." He adds that Mrs. Roth is past president of *Hadassah,* a woman's organization. Their daughter, Rachel, is religious and lives in an observant Orthodox community, keeps kosher, and does not drive or use the telephone on the Sabbath, from Friday sundown to Saturday after sundown.

Dr. Kelly asks Mr. Roth and Rachel if any resources in the Jewish community can help. Rachel says that she will contact Jewish Family and Children's Services for help with caregiver support and case management, and will ask members of *Hadassah* and the synagogue to visit and help with transportation and shopping.

Rachel adds that she is upset that her mother insists on being cremated, which is against Jewish law, particularly given the Holocaust when many Jews were incinerated. Dr. Kelly acknowledges this conflict and asks Rachel if a rabbi can help her deal with this issue.

At the follow-up visit the next month, Rachel reports that Jewish Family and Children's Services sent a nurse case manager (from their Seniors at Home program), who helped arrange for a lovely caregiver for Mrs. Roth. The nurse also helps with medication management, ensuring that the thyroid replacement hormone is given in the morning to help decrease night-time wandering. The Hebrew Free Loan program will help with finances. Rachel now visits once a month. She consulted with a community rabbi experienced with working with families from the full spectrum of religious observance. The rabbi acknowledged the conflict and the importance of Jewish *halachah* (law), noting that cremation violates the principle of respecting the body as sacred. He also acknowledged the centrality of the commandment to honor one's father and mother. Rachel is now more comfortable in honoring her mother's wishes, and talks with her father about finding a cemetery to bury her mother's ashes.

| CASE STUDY **2** | **Respecting Viewpoints of Family Decision Makers** |

Objectives
1. Understand Jewish views on end-of-life care, respiratory support, and do-not-resuscitate orders.
2. Reflect on your own values and beliefs regarding withdrawal of ventilator support and end-of-life care, and how this may influence how you care for patients.
3. Explore the challenges to compassion, understanding, and patience for health care professionals when a clinical situation is inherently conflicted, and the family's views may not reflect your own.

Mrs. Rubin is an 83-year-old Jewish widow who was admitted to the intensive care unit from the emergency department 10 days ago. She was at dinner with her daughter when her speech slurred, and she choked on some water and had a syncopal episode. Paramedics found her in respiratory distress, intubated her, and brought her to the emergency department. A CT scan showed a brainstem cerebrovascular accident (stroke). She remains intubated on a ventilator, opens her eyes, and can weakly squeeze her left hand on command. She has spontaneous respirations with inadequate ventilation but no gag reflex. When asked about an advance directive, her daughter Miriam says that her mother never wanted to talk about topics like this. Her mother used to say, "We go from strength to strength." Miriam says she cannot stand seeing her mother this way and feels that her mother would not want to be on a ventilator. The intensive care physician suggests that they continue treatment and see if her mother will recover.

Question:
1. What historical, cultural, or religious values may be involved in the daughter's decision-making process?

Mrs. Rubin's condition has not changed 10 days later. Dr. Thomas Roberts, Mrs. Rubin's primary care physician, meets with Miriam to discuss advance directives, and whether to place a tracheostomy and feeding tube or to withdraw respiratory support.

Miriam says, "I can't stand watching her this way. Mom has always been a very strong, active, and independent woman. I know that she would not want to live this way. But I just can't let her go. My mother is a Holocaust survivor from Hungary and has said that there is always hope, never give up." Miriam describes how her mother, as a teenager, was taken to a concentration camp along with four brothers, two sisters, parents, and grandparents. She was the only one to survive. After liberation in 1945, she moved to Israel, married, and moved to the United States in the late 1950s. She and her husband, who died several years ago, raised Miriam and a son, Jacob.

Miriam, herself a widow with two college-age children, has been taking care of "Mommy" every day. Jacob lives out of town and has little involvement with his mother's care.

Questions:
1. In a Jewish family, who might be involved in decision making?
2. What is the role of the rabbi or Jewish chaplain in medical decision making?

Dr. Roberts, whose personal decision would be to withdraw the ventilator and allow Mrs. Rubin to die, nonetheless wants to help Miriam come to a decision that is right for her and her mother. He suggests that Miriam speak with the hospital's Jewish chaplain. Miriam tells the chaplain of her anguish and conflict, and the pressure she feels from some members of the treatment team whom she overheard saying that they would never treat their own mother like this.

The chaplain explains there are different opinions in Jewish tradition in this situation. Some would continue providing care until the heart stops, whereas others would withdraw the ventilator so as to remove the obstacles to dying. He inquires about Mrs. Rubin's observance of Jewish tradition. Mrs. Rubin attended religious services on the high holidays at a local Orthodox synagogue. She lit Sabbath candles every Friday night and faithfully lit a candle in memory of her husband on the anniversary of his death. When Mr. Rubin was dying of lymphoma, the Rubins went to the Orthodox rabbi, whose advice Mrs. Rubin followed regarding medical treatments. When Mr. Rubin died, his body was prepared by the *Chevre Kaddisha*, the holy burial society, at the Jewish funeral home, and he was buried in a local Jewish cemetery. The chaplain suggests that Miriam consult with this same rabbi. The rabbi advises Miriam that she should not withdraw the ventilator because it was already initiated, and she should proceed with the tracheostomy and feeding tube. This was performed, and 1 week later Mrs. Rubin was discharged to a skilled nursing facility.

Mrs. Rubin is readmitted 3 months later with pneumonia and heart failure. She is off the ventilator, breathing room air through the tracheostomy, and being fed by a feeding tube. Sometimes, she opens her eyes to look at her daughter and moves her left hand nonpurposefully. Miriam tells Dr. Roberts that she had spoken with the rabbi, who said that Mrs. Rubin should not be placed on a ventilator again but should receive medicines for pneumonia and heart failure, as well as morphine for pain.

Miriam says she still cannot stand seeing her mother this way but cannot let her go. The Jewish chaplain visits regularly to provide emotional support and to offer prayers. Miriam complains that she heard one of the other physicians saying that she should "just let her go." Dr. Roberts explains to the medical team the importance of respecting the values and decisions of others. He acknowledges the daughter's devotion to her mother and the way she honors her mother.

Mrs. Rubin died 1 week later. Dr. Roberts was not able to attend the funeral, which he likes to do whenever possible. Instead, he visited the family at Mrs. Rubin's home 2 nights later during the *shiva* week of mourning after the funeral. Miriam thanked Dr. Roberts for his understanding and called him a *mentsch*, a person of kindness and integrity, for the way he helped Mrs. Rubin and for the *shiva* visit. For Dr. Roberts, the *shiva* visit helped create closure for himself.

Chaplain Bruce Feldstein, MD
Chaplain D'vorah Rose, RN, MA
Carol Hutner-Winograd, MD

References

About Jewish Healing. National Center for Jewish Healing. Available at: www.jewish-healing.org (accessed October 2006).

American Jewish Elderly and *Jewish Immigrants in the United States.* United Jewish Communities Special Reports. Available at: www.ujc.org/content_display. html?ArticleID=155417.

American Jews. Available at: http://www.answers.com/topic/american-jews#wp.

Cahill T. *The Gifts of the Jews—How a Tribe of Desert Nomads Changed the Way Everyone Thinks and Feels.* New York: Nan A. Talese/Anchor Books; 1998.

Dorff EN. *Matters of Life and Death—A Jewish Approach to Modern Medical Ethics.* Philadelphia: The Jewish Publication Society; 1998.

Eilberg A. Walking in the valley of the shadow: caring of the dying and their loved ones. In: Friedman DA (ed). *Jewish Pastoral Care: A Practical Handbook from Traditional and Contemporary Sources* (2nd ed). Woodstock, VT: Jewish Lights; 2005.

Friedman DA (ed). *Jewish Pastoral Care: A Practical Handbook from Traditional and Contemporary Sources* (2nd ed). Woodstock, VT: Jewish Lights; 2005.

Grollman EA. Death in Jewish Thought. In: Doka K, Morgan J (eds). *Death and Spirituality.* Amityville, NY: Baywood Publishing Co., Inc.; 1993:21–32.

Handler J, Hetherington K, Kelman S. *Give Me Your Hand. Traditional and Practical Guidance on Visiting the Sick* (2nd ed). Albany, CA: EKS; 1997.

Jewish Calendar. Available at: http://www.jewfaq.org/calendar.htm.

Jimena. Available at: http://www.jimena.org/index.htm.

Judaism. Available at: http://www.answers.com/Judaism.

Kashrut. Jewish Virtual Library. Available at: www.jewishvirtuallibrary.org/jsource/Judaism/kashrut.html.

Lamm M. *The Jewish Way in Death and Mourning.* New York: Jonathan David Publishers; 1969.

Levine E. Jewish views and customs on death. In: Parkes CM, Laungani A, Young B (eds). *Death and Bereavement Across Cultures.* New York: Routledge; 1997: 98–130.

Ozarowski J. *To Walk in God's Ways. Jewish Pastoral Perspectives on Illness and Bereavement.* Northvale, NJ: Jason Aronson; 1995.

Ponet JE. Reflections on mortality from a Jewish perspective. In: Spiro, Curren, Wandel (eds). *Facing Death.* New Haven, CT: Yale University Press; 1996: 129–136.

Riemer J, Stampfer N (eds). *So That Your Values Live On: Ethical Wills and How to Prepare Them.* Woodstock, VT: Jewish Lights; 1991.

Schacter-Shalomi Z, Miller RS. *From Age-ing to Sage-ing: A Profound New Vision of Growing Older.* New York: Warner Books; 1995.

Shapiro RM. *Last Breaths: A Guide to Easing Another's Dying.* Miami, FL: Temple Beth Or; 1993.

Silberman J. Jewish spiritual care in the acute care hospital. In: Friedman DA (ed). *Jewish Pastoral Care: A Practical Handbook from Traditional and Contemporary Sources* (2nd ed). Woodstock, VT: Jewish Lights; 2005.

Timeline for the History of Judaism. Available at: www.jewishvirtuallibrary.org/jsource/
History/timeline.html.
United States Census 2000. Available at: www.census.gov/prod/2001pubs/c2kbr01-10.
pdf.
World Religions: Judaism. Available at: http://endlink.lurie.northwestern.edu/religion_
spirituality/judaism.htm.

Additional Resources

Judaism and Health, Aging, Dying, and Death

Bay Area Jewish Healing Center
www.jewishhealingcenter.org/

Brener A. *Mourning and Mitzvah: A Guided Journal for Walking the Mourner's Path
Through Grief to Healing.* Woodstock, VT: Jewish Lights; 1993.

EndLink-Resource for End-of-Life Care Education
http://endlink.lurie.northwestern.edu/

Hiddur: The Center for Aging and Judaism
www.rrc.edu

Jewish Holidays Calendar
http://ujc.org/content_display.html?ArticleID=69770

Jewish Medical Directives for Health Care
http://www.rabbinicalassembly.org/docs/medical%20directives.pdf

Kalsman Institute on Judaism and Health
www.huc.edu/kalsman/

National Center for Jewish Healing
www.jewishhealing.org/

Ritual Well
www.ritualwell.org/

Jewish Community Resources

Association of Jewish Aging Services
  www.ajas.org/

Association of Jewish Family and Children's Agencies
  www.ajfca.org/

Hebrew Immigrant Aid Society
  www.hias.org

International Association of Hebrew Free Loans
  www.freeloan.org/

Jewish Community Centers Association of America
  www.jcca.org/

National Association of Jewish Chaplains
  www.najc.org/

CHAPTER 8

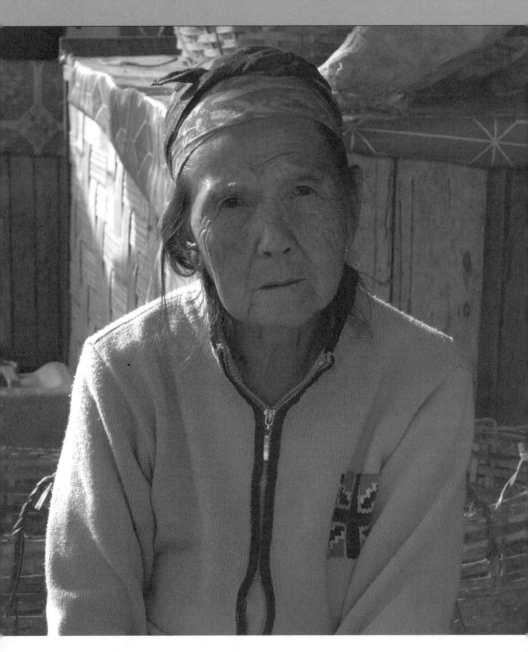

Shamanism: Its Practice among Hmong Americans

The practice of shamanism, which originated in the indigenous cultures of Siberia and Central Asia, dates back over 25,000 years and is the oldest form of healing. The shaman is an expert in working in the spiritual realm and with human souls, and he or she uses trance to mediate between the physical and spiritual worlds. Through trance, a shaman is able to see and navigate in the spirit world. Rituals often include chanting; dancing, jumping, or another form of movement; or drumming to enter the trance state. The community to which the shaman belongs believes that the shaman has special powers to heal the sick.

The shaman is an expert in working in the spiritual realm and with human souls, and he or she uses trance to mediate between the physical and spiritual worlds.

The shaman's main task is to identify when a soul has left a person's body and to return it. Evil demons, sorcerers, or spirits of deceased family members may capture a soul. The shaman has the power to diagnose the problem and negotiate appropriate interventions for return of the missing soul to the human body. Shamanic practice is still an integral part of many cultural groups around the world. Although there are similarities in all shamanic practices, each culture has developed its own unique beliefs that set them apart.

Shamanic practice is still an integral part of many cultural groups around the world.

Hmong traditional healers, known as *txiv neeb*, are extremely important individuals in the Hmong community. The word *shaman* is the English word often used to describe this group of healers. For centuries, Hmong shamans have held positions of spiritual, religious, and political leadership in their communities. Many were also expert herbalists. Until the Vietnam War era, Hmong shamans provided most of the health services available to the Hmong population residing in remote villages in the mountains of Laos.

The Hmong were self-sufficient farmers, isolated from the rest of the world. Because no doctors were available for people in the villages, the Hmong language does not have an equivalent word for "doctor."

In Hmong, it takes three words to describe what a doctor does: *kws kho mob* (skill, take care, illness). After the 1960s, many Hmong began using the English word "doctor."

Most Hmong patients and their families who do not speak English lack a framework within which to understand how a physician makes a diagnosis and recommends treatment.

Most Hmong patients and their families who do not speak English lack a framework within which to understand how a physician makes a diagnosis and recommends treatment. They have been isolated from the major historical developments of modern medicine. Because they lack knowledge and understanding of concepts such as germ theory of disease, antisepsis, scientific method, surgery, and preventive health, Hmong people lack both conceptual comprehension and language equivalents.

Most health professionals today assume that patients have at least a basic understanding about medical technology—from basic tools of examination, such as the stethoscope, to more advanced diagnostic tools, such as an electrocardiograph or medical imaging techniques, to common medical or surgical procedures, such as anesthesia or a blood transfusion. The Hmong patient may not possess this understanding. Because Hmong patients rely on their world knowledge and previous life experiences to make medical decisions, it is important for physicians to try to link new medical information to Hmong spiritual life experiences.

Immigration History

Beginning in the early 1960s, the Hmong way of life was abruptly changed. The US Central Intelligence Agency recruited Hmong to fight the communist Pathet Lao troops. These troops had invaded the northern provinces of Laos where the Hmong lived. The Hmong were one of several ethnic groups in northern Laos who wanted to maintain their independent lifestyle and were willing to fight for their freedom. The Central Intelligence Agency trained and supported Hmong for covert operations. During this time, Hmong families forced to abandon their villages became dependent on food and supplies dropped from the air. For more than 10 years, the Hmong held out against the North Vietnamese soldiers. The United States did not want their covert operations to become public knowledge, thus the name the "secret war" of Laos. The Hmong helped the US government avoid sending

American troops into this neutral country and helped to rescue many American pilots shot down by the North Vietnamese.

After the United States withdrew troops from the region, communists overthrew the royal Lao government in 1975. One-third of the Hmong in Laos died during and after the war, and another third fled to Thailand. Most of those who became refugees in Thailand resettled in the United States, France, Australia, or French Guiana from 1975 to 1997. About 15,000 of the Hmong refugees who remained in Thailand at a Buddhist Temple (Wat Tham Krabok) were recently resettled to the United States during 2004–2006. Almost all of these recent refugees practice "old" religion and rely on shamans.

Today, approximately 200,000–250,000 Hmong people live in the United States. Between 60% and 70% (percentage varies by geographic region) practice their "old" traditional religion called *Coj Dab* and rely on Hmong shamans. Although it is difficult to estimate how many Hmong shamans actively practice in the United States, in Laos a small village of five families would usually have one shaman. Over 100 known shamans practice in one central California community with a Hmong population of about 8,000. About two-thirds of these shamans are men, and one-third women.

> *Today, approximately 200,000–250,000 Hmong people live in the United States.*

Gender Considerations

Male and female shamans are evaluated by the community based on their ability to heal. Some develop better reputations than others. Families often seek shamans based on their reputation; gender alone is not a criterion used for decisions.

Religious Basis for Views of Health and Disease

Chinese scholars wrote the first record of Hmong civilization in 2679 BCE. From centuries of Chinese influence, aspects of Confucianism, Taoism, Animism, and Shamanism intertwine together to form the Hmong religious and spiritual belief system. The physical world (life on earth), the spiritual world (otherworld), and the heaven (high place in sky where souls reincarnate and return to earth) are important realms.

Beliefs About Death and Life After Death

Traditional Hmong believe that life is a cycle of birth and rebirth. The physical and spiritual worlds are equally important. Spirits in people,

Traditional Hmong believe that life is a cycle of birth and rebirth. The physical and spiritual worlds are equally important.

animals, and inanimate objects are interdependent and can directly affect the health and well-being of a Hmong person and his or her family. Hmong are cautious about surgery. Few Hmong have received organ transplants, and it is very rare for them to consent to organ donation. Traditional Hmong worry about possible consequences that they may have in the next life after reincarnation.

The Hmong believe that a person has several souls. There is no consistent agreement on the number of souls that a person has; some traditions say 3, and others as many as 32. Practices within the 18 Hmong clans have distinct variations.

Belief in spirits affects every aspect of daily Hmong life and is the basis for Hmong healing traditions, health-promoting ceremonies, and rituals. A person's souls and physical body must function in harmony as a single integrated unit to experience spiritual, mental, and physical health. When there is an imbalance, illness results. One aspect of the imbalance may include *poob plig,* "loss of soul." This concept lacks equivalent meaning and any associated treatment in biomedicine.

Spiritual disease and healing are critical concepts in the Hmong community.

However, spiritual disease and healing are critical concepts in the Hmong community. Shamanism and the essential source of healing it provides for Hmong are poorly understood by Western health care providers and health educators.

Healing and Health-Promoting Ceremonies and Rituals

The Hmong New Year ceremonies celebrated in November and December in the United States are important for the health and well-being of Hmong families. The first Hmong shaman, *Shee Yee,* defeated an evil spirit that destroyed Hmong people. The New Year's ceremony (*Nkaum Toj* or *Lwm sub)* celebrates Hmong freedom from the evil spirit.

The ceremony is led by a shaman and involves "throwing away the old" and bad part of the current year's experiences and bringing in the new life for the next year. Family members walk under a new year's pole and woven green grass rope three times forward and three times backward.

After returning home, each family demonstrates filial piety with a soul calling (*hu plig)* ceremony. A soul caller or the head of household conducts this ceremony for his own family. Early on the first day of the new year, the family honors the elders and ancestors with the ceremony *pe tsiab*.

The New Year's ceremonies protect the family in the upcoming year. Preventive medicine is a concept that has a parallel in the New Year's ceremonies, because the goal is to protect individuals from health problems in the future.

> *The New Year's ceremonies protect the family in the upcoming year.*

Hmong shamans do not choose to become healers. They are instead "chosen" by the *neeb* spirit. Healing is a vocation. To be self-sufficient in the United States, most shamans need to have an additional occupation. In contrast, physicians, nurses, and other health professionals choose to pursue a career in medicine, nursing, or other discipline. For some health professionals, healing is a vocational calling as well as an occupation.

Pa Lor, a new shaman, describes her own experience of being chosen to become a shaman with an initiatory 5 years of illness by the *neeb* spirit. She reports that none of the biomedical care she obtained from physicians and chiropractors for leg and stomach pains resulted in a definitive diagnosis or cure. Her illness culminated with a desolate feeling one night that she was "going to die." Her frightened mother called a shaman for assistance. As soon as the shamanic ritual started, her family was astonished as they watched her mimic the shaman's movements while she sat with her eyes closed on the couch. Pa recalls her inability to control her body movements during the ritual. The performing shaman diagnosed Pa's problem and notified the *neeb* spirit that Pa would accept the calling even though she never obtained permission or agreement from Pa. Eighty-nine collected biographies and similar experiences of being chosen of Hmong shamans have been documented in the Partners in Healing project in Merced, California.

Hmong believe that a *neeb* spirit will choose only people that are righteous, honest, and trustworthy, and exhibit human kindness toward others. The act of being chosen requires that the person make a life-long commitment to being a healer. This includes the responsibility to be accessible to those requesting services. Even though most shamans provide services exclusively to Southeast Asian refugees, they

> *The act of being chosen requires that the person make a life-long commitment to being a healer.*

state that they are available to any person regardless of race, ethnicity, or gender. In central California, there are only a few anecdotal reports of mainstream Americans using the services of a shaman.

Hmong shamans also accept certain dietary restrictions. Eating restricted foods can cause severe gastrointestinal problems. Shamans understand that negotiating for spiritual health can be personally dangerous and may even cause their own death. Similar to Western health professionals, Hmong shamans begin the treatment process by diagnosing and determining the etiology of health problems. The shaman, however, assesses the "soul status" or *ua neeb saib* and then provides treatment by negotiating with the spirit(s) causing the illness.

Hmong shamans do not receive formal instruction or supervision. Usually a master shaman is identified to help the newly chosen shaman learn numerous details of shamanic practice, such as setting up an altar (*teeb thaj neeb*). The master may be asked questions about particular cases, but he or she does not train or educate regarding how to heal. The *neeb* spirit calls each shaman and provides knowledge about spiritual practices over time. These "spirit helpers" provide direction to the newly chosen shaman during trance. Pa Lor knows her three spirit helpers by first name. She reports that additional spirit helpers will come to help when she is ready.

> *Some Hmong shamans specialize in a particular health condition that is usually related to the illness that they experienced when chosen.*

Some Hmong shamans specialize in a particular health condition that is usually related to the illness that they experienced when chosen. Services are provided in patients' homes. In this respect, the practice of the Hmong shamans is comparable to that of the general practitioner of the 19th and early 20th century. Older Americans in the United States have reported the significance of a physician's home visit to treat a medical condition. In a recent study of shaman satisfaction, Hmong families were more satisfied when a shaman conducted ceremonies in their own homes rather than from an alternative location.

The goal of a Hmong shaman's treatment is to cure a patient's health problem by negotiating *(pauj dab – hloov ntsuj plig)* for the person's soul. This might involve offering gifts such as joss paper and joss sticks *(nyiaj txiag xyab ntaws)* and/or exchanging the soul of an animal for the soul of the sick person. Negotiation strategies include a variety of ways to outwit or fool the spirit into giving up the person's soul. Great risk is involved in this negotiation process. There are numerous narrative stories about shamans who died during or immediately after negotiations when overpowering spirits prevailed and seized their souls.

A Hmong shaman never provides a 100% guarantee. He or she agrees to provide 100% of their skill and effort to cure the spiritual cause of the health problem. Similarly, physicians can reassure a Hmong family that they will do everything possible to help their loved one but cannot provide a 100% guarantee. Exploratory surgery, medication trial, and/or medication adjustments can be compared with the different ways that a shaman determines the cause of the problem and/or success of the shamanic intervention.

Sacred Objects

Divination rituals prevent rivalry among shamans. These rituals help families decide which Hmong shaman will be the best one to help a particular patient. An egg that maintains its balance on a bottle indicates that a particular shaman may be able to resolve the problem. The identified shaman will also use a buffalo horn split into two matching pieces; when the pieces are clicked together and dropped onto the floor, they land in a variety of possible combinations that correspond to different situations. The positioning indicates if the shaman has the right combination of experience and skill to help, and if the spirit(s) of the shaman will be strong enough to retrieve the missing soul. Although the technology differs greatly, health professionals can refer to this when they describe various tests and tools used to determine a patient's diagnosis or to identify the specialist best able to treat that particular problem.

Hmong shamans often wait 3 days after their initial diagnostic ritual to evaluate patient improvement before intervening (spirits willing to negotiate) or concluding with a healing ceremony. They are more concerned about health and wellness than about the patient's illness. This is helpful to remember when explaining treatment recommendations for chronic illness. If a patient does not show improvement, the shaman is not blamed. The explanation may be that the evil spirits are back or are more powerful than the intervention provided by a particular shaman.

> If a patient does not show improvement, the shaman is not blamed.

The rhythmical beating of the bronze gong (*nruas neeb*) summons the *neeb* spirit and is used to rally spirits during the ceremony. Its reverberating, penetrating sound symbolizes spiritual power, and it serves as a shield to protect the shaman. A Hmong assistant—the shaman's husband, wife, mother, father, son, or other close family member—continues beating as directed until the journey into the spirit world ends. Hmong shamans must have assistance during a particular ritual or ceremony to ensure their own physical safety while in trance. In addition, other members of a patient's family serve in a variety of established roles that assist and support the overall healing process. Similarly, most surgeries require a second physician to assist during the surgery. Many other health professionals serve in designated helping roles. In many health settings today, members of a variety of disciplines work together as a team to provide patient-centered care.

A black, red, or white hood or veil *(daim thi hauv)* covers the face and eyes of a Hmong shaman during trance. Some say that this allows shamans to focus on the inner vision that they use to "see" into the spiritual world. Others report that it helps to keep the malevolent spirits from recognizing the shamans' faces when they return to the physical human world. Other essential tools include a spiritual sword *(ntaj neeb)*, an iron hoop or cymbal with pieces of round metal attachments that is rattled *(txiab neeb)* such as the harness of a symbolic horse, finger bell rings *(tswb neeb)* used to hit evil spirits, and a wooden bench *(rooj neeb)* that symbolizes a winged horse.

Each shaman builds his or her own altar at home.

Each shaman builds his or her own altar at home. Although some pieces are standard, they all look unique. A bowl of water symbolizing the dragon's pool at the cave of Shee Yee is an important piece. A candle on the altar lights the way to the spirit world. A saucer of rice with an egg in the center and three sticks of incense serves as a food offering to the special *neeb* spirit of the shaman. Usually, there are three small containers with water, tea, and rice wine for the spirits. There may also be a container of puffed corn for the symbolic horse. Similarly, health professionals use a variety of different tools based on their practice specialty.

Chants during trance communicate with the spirits. Chinese words are incorporated as needed. Pa Lor reports that she speaks other languages such as Lao, Chinese, and Khmer when she chants during trance. Some spirits are frightened when they hear words in different languages. During trance, spiritual helpers make themselves available, and spiritual armies mobilize to assist the shaman.

A newly chosen shaman may be closer to the spirits. They report feeling more controlled by their helper spirit(s) than in control of the spirit(s). Many Hmong patients are therefore concerned about the age of health professionals. For example, resident physicians and student nurses assigned to Hmong patients may not be trusted as much as an older health professional, who is perceived as being wiser through experience. It is helpful to describe the advantage that individuals in training have in regards to the most current knowledge base.

Many Hmong patients are therefore concerned about the age of health professionals.

Hmong shamans do not charge for services unless it is determined that their intervention has cured the patient. Hmong patients often have difficulty understanding the concept of medical payments when the patient has not been cured. Usually, the family of the ill person incurs the costs for the healing ceremony. Negotiation may include promise of the exchange of an animal's soul for the release of a human soul. Often, a specific animal is purchased for sacrifice. The animal chosen might be a chicken, pig, cow, or goat, depending on the situation; the need for a duck or other animal is rare. Treating an animal reverently is important, and an expert kills it quickly to minimize suffering. Although this aspect of shamanism is its most controversial practice in the United States, it is important to understand the Hmong perspective. In the villages, meat was not part of the daily diet. During healing ceremonies, the animal sacrificed provided nourishment to the patient and extended family. Ceremonies brought the community together to show collective caring. The large number of people who come to demonstrate their support of a particular patient surprises physicians who observe Hmong healing ceremonies.

In the United States, most city ordinances prohibit animal sacrifice. It is acceptable to butcher animals for human consumption only in approved slaughterhouses. Animals "give" their lives to benefit people in scientific laboratories. A Hmong shaman that visited the University of California–Davis laboratory quickly made the parallel between animals used in scientific studies and animals sacrificed in healing rituals.

Families usually reward the shaman in some way for a successful soul retrieval, which may include up to $300 for a lengthy, complicated healing ceremony.

Families also purchase items such as incense *(xyab)* that must be burned, spirit money called joss paper *(ntawv nyiaj)*, and materials to build a temporary altar. Families usually reward the shaman in some way for a successful soul retrieval, which may include up to $300 for a lengthy, complicated healing ceremony. The purchase of needed medical supplies or medications can be associated with shaman compensation.

Although the Hmong do not identify or name Confucianism as an integral part of their belief system, maintaining spiritual health requires honoring ancestors, as in Confucianism. Conducting regular ceremonies that demonstrate respect for ancestors and recently deceased family members help the Hmong retain cultural connections with past, present, and future generations. Prosperity, health, happiness, and longevity are linked to honoring ancestors. The head of household performs rituals at home.

Views on Do-Not-Resuscitate Orders, Nutrition, and Hydration at End of Life

> *Filial piety is important at the end of life. In general, the Hmong want everything possible done for their loved one.*

Filial piety is important at the end of life. In general, the Hmong want everything possible done for their loved one. Most are not familiar with procedures such as cardiopulmonary resuscitation, intubation, or artificial ventilation. Nutrition and hydration is expected, and families are especially concerned when patients are unable to consume Hmong staples, such as rice and chicken soup.

Religious Customs and Rituals for Dying Patients and After Death

Immediate and extended family members visit a dying patient to pay their respects. Life after death is an important concept. Many important rituals are associated with preparing and dressing the body. It is important to dress the deceased person in special clothing made for him or her. During the 3- to 10-day funeral, relatives must stay with the body day and night. An expert plays the *qeej*, an important musical instrument made from bamboo, to guide the soul of the deceased on its journey to the ancestors. Collectively, individuals mourn the loss of the deceased by crying loudly at designated times during the funeral. There are many duties in managing a Hmong funeral. Some women cook rice, a group of men butcher and cook animals, and others are designated to oversee other important tasks. Relatives also make monetary contributions to defray the funeral costs.

Summary

The religious traditions of the Hmong provide individual patients and their families with their own ethical foundation for medical decision making. Hmong patients rely on a range of cultural and spiritual beliefs that provide a context for meaning, purpose, and hope during times of illness. Shamanism provides an important therapeutic support system to help them cope. Understanding the traditional Hmong spirituality and "old" religion will help to build trust and ultimately improve the effectiveness and outcome of clinical practice. Patient-centered care involves demonstrating respect for Hmong spiritual beliefs and practices.

CASE STUDY **1**	**Accommodating Cultural Religious Practices with Respect and Flexibility**

> ### Objectives
> 1. Discuss how spiritual beliefs influence a Hmong family's end-of-life decision making.
> 2. Discuss how a Hmong shaman can complement provided medical care.

You practice family medicine in an ethnically diverse county in central California. After a busy afternoon in the primary care clinic, you receive a call from a nurse in the intensive care unit. She reports that a patient's condition continues to deteriorate and that the patient remains a "full code." She also mentions that the family is waiting to speak with the patient.

Mr. Her is a 65-year-old Hmong refugee from Laos who has lived in the United States for 20 years and is a respected leader of a large Hmong clan. Now comatose in the intensive care unit, Mr. Her had for several days postponed consenting to exploratory surgery because the surgeon did not offer a conclusive diagnosis. Because of prolonged exposure to lethal toxins from a gangrenous bowel, he is not expected to survive. He has 11 major complications, including septicemia, acute renal failure, respiratory failure, and seizures.

Mr. Her's son, wife, and 15 other family members are sitting in a crowded waiting room. Other Hmong people stand in the hallway. As you enter the room, Hmong voices hush. They wait for news about Mr. Her's condition, hoping to hear that he will improve. In broken English, you learn that Mr. Her has brothers who have come from Minnesota and France.

Question:
1. How might an understanding of filial piety help with the family discussions about end-of-life decisions, such as do-not-resuscitate orders?

Koua Her, the patient's oldest son, often serves as the family interpreter. He struggles to interpret medical information to the family, so you request a trained Hmong interpreter. When the interpreter arrives, you briefly share the purpose of the family meeting. Through the interpreter, you introduce the Hmong interpreter and explain that she will interpret all information accurately. You state that Mr. Her's condition is worsening and that he may not live longer than 1–2 days.

You acknowledge that you and other staff respect the family and community demonstration of love, caring, and support of Mr. Her during this time of serious illness. You explain that in this country, it is important for the doctor to discuss with the family what Mr. Her would want the medical staff to do if his heart stops beating. You state that Mr. Her is no longer able to breathe on his own without the help of a machine. His kidneys have stopped working, and he needs hemodialysis. Special doctors do not expect him to get better. If his heart stops beating, doctors and nurses would press down on his chest many times to squeeze his heart to try to get it to beat again. This is very painful and is not usually successful when a person is in very poor condition. The family listens carefully and asks questions. The son says that they will discuss it together to make their decision. They express their gratitude.

Question:
1. How might an understanding of Hmong shamanism help you and the hospital provide culturally sensitive care?

Before leaving the family meeting, the patient's brother requests your permission to allow a Hmong *neeb* (shaman) to perform a ceremony in the hospital. You inquire about the shaman's ceremony. The brother directs the question to the shaman also sitting in the room. He explains that he will perform magic healing and a string-tying ceremony. When asked about magic healing, he describes sprinkling spiritual water over Mr. Her's body. He states that the string-tying ceremony involves chanting when a red string is tied around Mr. Her's neck.

You explain that Mr. Her has several open abdominal wounds and a tracheostomy. You make clear the need to use sterile gloves and sterile water. The shaman agrees to modify the ceremony and use the special water provided by the hospital. You state that a nurse will help him with the gloves and water. You also ask if the string can be placed on Mr. Her's wrist, as you have seen on many other Hmong patients. The shaman explains that because Mr. Her's problem is so serious, the string must be tied around his neck. You state that a nurse will need to supervise the string tying and ensure that this string is securely taped to the patient's neck to prevent it from interfering with tracheostomy care. The shaman agrees.

Several nurses supervise the ceremony. One nurse documents that Mr. Her opened his eyes during the ceremony for the first time. Later that day, he followed basic commands. Over the next 4 weeks, his condition improved remarkably. The shaman conducted several additional healing ceremonies under nursing supervision during the patient's hospital stay.

After a short stay in a local rehabilitation facility, Mr. Her walks in to see you for a follow-up clinic appointment. He thanks you for the help that you and the other doctors provided to him and invites you to a community gathering in his honor.

In this case, there was a miraculous full recovery. However, if Mr. Her had not survived, the fact that you, the physician, and the hospital respected the family's request to conduct healing ceremonies would have eliminated the possibility that something more might have been offered to heal him. The culturally responsive care that was provided will be shared within the informal but extensive communication network of the Hmong community.

Pa Lor, Hmong Neeb (Shaman)
Marilyn Mochel, RN

References and Additional Resources

Brown WS, Murphy N, Newton Maloney H (eds). *Whatever Happened to the Soul? Scientific and Theological Portraits of Human Nature.* Minneapolis, MN: Fortress Press; 1998.

Conquergood D. *I'm a Shaman, a Hmong Life Story with Ethnographic Commentary.* Center for Urban and Regional Affairs, University of Minnesota, 1986.

Culhane-Pera K, et al. *Healing by Heart: Clinical and Ethical Case Stories of Hmong Familes and Western Providers.* Nashville: Vanderbilt University Press; 2003.

Fadiman A. *The Spirit Catches You and You Fall Down: A Hmong Child, Her American Doctors, and the Collision of Two Cultures.* New York: The Noonday Press; 1997.

Helsel D, Mochel M, Bauer R. Shamans in a Hmong American Community. *J Altern Complement Med* 2004;10(6):933–938.

Her C, Culhane-Pera K. Culturally responsive care for Hmong patients. *Postgrad Med* 2004;116(6):39–42, 45–46.

Hmong Shamanism. In: Barnes L, Sered SS (eds). *Religion and Healing in America.* Oxford, England: Oxford University Press; 2005:439–454.

Inclusion of Indigenous and Traditional Knowledge and Social Capital in the Community-based Participatory Research Aspect of Heritable Disorders and Genetic Diseases in Newborns and Children. Advisory Committee on Heritable Disorders and Genetic Diseases in Newborns and Children, Washington, DC; 2004.

Kleinman A, Eisenberg E, Good B. Culture, illness and care: clinical lessons from anthropologic and cross-cultural research. *Ann Intern Med* 1978;888:251–258.

Pinzon-Perez H, Moua N, Perez MA. Understanding satisfaction with shamanic practices among the Hmong in rural California. *Intl Electr J Health Educ* (www.iejhe.org) 2005;8:18–23.

Plotnikoff GA, Numerich C, Wu C, Yang D, Phua X. Hmong shamanism: animist spiritual healing in Minnesota. *Minnesota Med* 2002;85(6):29–34.

Split Horn: *The Life of a Hmong Shaman in America*. Director: Taggart Siegel; 2001.

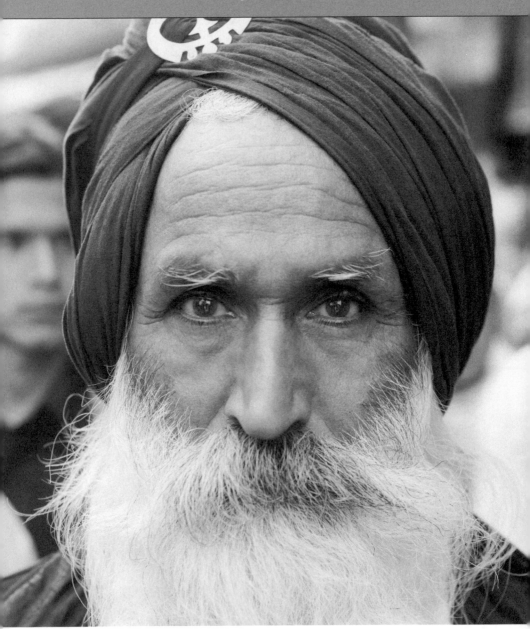

CHAPTER 9

Sikhism

Sikhism is the fifth largest organized religion (22 million) in the world but is still not very well known. Therefore, the peculiarities of health care as it relates to Sikhs (followers of Sikhism) are understood even less. Old age is much respected in the faith, and mutual respect is at the core of relationships. Sikhs value empathy and a caring nature in their providers.

Sikhism was founded in 1499 by Guru Nanek in the northwest part of India in the state of Punjab; therefore, Sikhs are sometimes called Punjabis. The teachings of Sikhism are based on the writings of Guru Nanek and nine other gurus who succeeded him, the last of whom lived in the 17th century.

> *Sikhism was founded in 1499 by Guru Nanek in the northwest part of India in the state of Punjab.*

In America, Sikhs are widely dispersed but live in much larger concentrations in New York, New Jersey, California, and New Mexico.

Preferred Cultural Terms and Religious Beliefs

The fundamental belief of Sikhs is that there is only One, Universal, Formless, Timeless God of all the people, Who is also the creator of this universe and all living beings. *Sikh* means *disciple*, and Sikhism is a path of discipline by meditating on God's name, earning a living by honest means, sharing good fortunes with the needy, and serving humanity selflessly.

Baptized Sikhs, also known as *Khalsa*, wear on their person at all times five religious symbols that are articles of faith. These symbols are known as the "five Ks" because their names start with the letter "K":

1. Uncut hair *(Kesh)*, a gift from God representing spirituality
2. A wooden comb *(Kangha)*, symbolizing cleanliness
3. A steel bracelet *(Kara)*, representing self-restraint and link to God
4. A short sword *(Kirpaan)*, an emblem of courage and commitment to truth and justice
5. A type of underwear knickers *(Kachhehra)*, representing purity of moral character

The religious significance of the headdress (a turban for men or a scarf for women) should be respected, because it is a covering for one of the five Ks *(Kesh)* and is also a symbol of a Sikh's honor.

Generally, practicing Sikhs do not cut their hair and do not consume tobacco products, alcohol, intoxicants, or other illicit drugs.

Sikhs believe that whosoever is born has eventually to die. The physical body is perishable, but the soul is eternal.

Sikhs believe that whosoever is born has eventually to die. The physical body is perishable, but the soul is eternal. The soul is a part of God, and it longs for reunion with the Supreme Being. Liberation from the cycle of birth and death, from millions of life forms, is the basis of the Sikh understanding of the purpose of life. Human life is the gift of the Divine, and its termination is a return to the Divine source.

Priests in the Sikh traditions are called *Granthi* and read from the Holy Scriptures, the *Guru Granth Sahib.* A Granthi is also a spiritual leader, a religious counselor, a teacher, and a role model. Granthi also perform the religious ceremonies and conduct Sunday meetings in the *Gurdwara*, the Sikh temple. They are expected to be especially accomplished in classical music and traditionally sing many of the scriptures while they accompany themselves on a musical instrument *(Dhillon).*

Formality of Address

Male Sikhs have the last or middle name "Singh," which means "lion" and indicates their roots in bravery and to protect the weak and oppressed. Female Sikhs have the middle or last name "Kaur," which means "princess." Thus, the proper terms of address are Mr. Singh and Mrs. Kaur.

Sikhs give much respect to their elders. They also hold physicians in high regard.

Sikhs give much respect to their elders. They also hold physicians in high regard. They call their doctor "sahib" (meaning *master* or *sir*, a term of much respect). They call nurses "sister," which is also a term of respect.

Language and Literacy

The common language is Punjabi. Many Sikhs are well educated and can converse in English. Some older adults may not speak English; others may understand it if spoken slowly in short, simple sentences. However, they may not be able to express subtle details and may require assistance from Punjabi or Hindi interpreters. Most of the time, some-one who speaks and understands English will accompany older Sikhs to a doctor's visit.

Effective Communication

Traditionally, older Sikh adults prefer their physician to be in charge and in control. They want him or her to make decisions and tell them what to do. If a physician shows signs of uncertainty or wants to leave the decision making to the patient, it could be interpreted as ineptness or a sign of medical incompetence.

Some older adults may not be satisfied with explanations that symptoms can be caused by viral illnesses and will likely be self-limited, and that antibiotics are not needed. They are generally looking for a prescription or a pill when they visit their physician.

Older Sikhs are relationship-oriented. They love to talk about family members if they feel comfortable with the physician. Sometimes, because of this, it is considered rude or even disrespectful if the medical visit is ended abruptly so that the physician can stay on time. The best approach is to always explain the follow-up plan to bring the visit to a close.

Older Sikhs are relationship-oriented. They love to talk about family members if they feel comfortable with the physician.

Tradition and Health Beliefs

Family Structure and Relationship

The family is the basic and most important social unit.

- The man is the head of the family; authority lines are from the father to the oldest son, who is responsible for the welfare of the entire family, including extended family.
- Older parents are respected and looked after by the son's family.
- Children are expected to respect, listen to, and obey parents, older siblings, and family members. Girls are expected to stay with parents until they get married.
- Sikh families value education and high academic achievement. Children generally are not expected to do household chores. Parents would rather see their children spend time on studying. Parents pay tuition fees for college or university education.

- Although numbers of cross-cultural marriages are increasing, arranged marriages are still prevalent in the South Asian community.

Diet and Nutrition

Many Sikhs are vegetarians. Their staple foods are *roti* (flat bread), rice, *daals* (grains, legumes, and pulses), fruits, and vegetables. Food prepared with chicken broth, eggs, or fish and other seafood is still considered non-vegetarian. Some Sikhs do eat chicken, fish, goat, or lamb meat but avoid beef because of cultural reasons. Sikhs do not eat any ritual meat. Eating vegetarian or non-vegetarian meals is an individual preference. If there are no dietary restrictions, the patient may be asked his or her food preferences, or food can be brought from home. Sikhs do not fast for any religious reason.

> *Sikhs do not fast for any religious reason.*

Food items are considered to have hot or cold qualities. This concept means that certain food items have a hot or cold impact on the body. For example, nuts, eggs, papaya, mango, and eggplant are considered hot foods. Examples of cold foods are melon, rice, cilantro, and buttermilk. Sikhs try to avoid eating milk and yogurt together or eating fish with milk.

> *The sanctity of life is an injunction, and human life is of the highest form.*

General Beliefs and Practices

The sanctity of life is an injunction, and human life is of the highest form.

- Blood transfusions are allowed.
- Assisted suicide and euthanasia are not encouraged.
- Maintaining a terminal patient on artificial life support for a prolonged period in a vegetative state is not encouraged.
- Organ transplantation, both donating and receiving, is allowed.
- Autopsy is permitted.
- Genetic engineering to cure a disease is acceptable. To date, Sikhs are opposed to human cloning.
- Male infants are not circumcised.

Medical and Nursing Care

An essential aspect of health care is the role of the health care provider in understanding the concerns of the patient and family and communicating those concerns to all those involved in the decision-making process. This includes comforting patients and consoling their family members so that they can accept the disease state, and if possible, taking care of the family's needs beyond the medical aspects.

Principles used by ethicists include preservation of the patient's faith, the sanctity of life, alleviation of suffering, respect for the patient's autonomy while providing the best available medical treatment without causing undue harm, and always being honest and truthful in giving information.

Important Aspects in Care

Suggestions for health care providers in caring for an older Sikh patient include the following:

- Respect modesty and privacy (eg, knock on the door, announce your arrival).
- Do not interrupt a praying patient for routine care.
- Respect the patient's personal space by limiting unnecessary touching.
- Be sensitive to the significance of the five Ks (religious symbols or articles of faith), which Sikhs may be wearing on their person at all times. After removing their headdress, Sikh patients may want to keep their head covered with an alternative, such as a small turban or scarf. (A surgical bouffant cap is acceptable.) The headdress should be respected; if removed, it should be given to the family or placed with the patient's personal belongings. The patient's headdress should not be placed with their shoes.
- Consult the patient or family before shaving or removing hair from any part of the patient's body. This applies to both male and female patients.

Other Practices

Sikh women may insist on covering their bodies with more than a hospital gown. They may also request that, when possible, examinations be done with the gown on.

Although Sikhism does not ban treatment from being provided by a practitioner of the opposite sex, a same-sex practitioner is preferred, especially if the patient requests it.

Cleanliness is part of the Sikh way of life. Daily bathing and personal hygiene care should be provided unless advised otherwise by the attending physician because of a medical reason. Washing and conditioning of hair, including male facial hair, with shampoo or soap should be done as frequently as needed. Hair can be dried naturally or with an electric hair dryer. At a minimum, hair should be combed daily.

Daily bathing and personal hygiene care should be provided unless advised otherwise by the attending physician because of a medical reason.

It is a Sikh cultural and religious practice to visit the sick. Hospital and nursing home staff should be open and understanding of visits by family members, including children, and friends, when practical.

Culture-Specific Health Risks

Sikh older adults have an increased risk of dyslipidemia, especially high triglycerides and low HDL. This may be related to their dietary habits of eating fried food and foods cooked in saturated fats.

Older Sikh adults have an increased risk of developing diabetes because of genetics, central obesity, dyslipidemia, and poor dietary habits.

Older Sikh adults have an increased risk of developing diabetes because of genetics, central obesity, dyslipidemia, and poor dietary habits. They also love sweets, which can interfere with good control of diabetes. They are also at risk of poorly controlled hypertension because of high salt consumption. All of these risk factors translate into an increased risk of coronary artery disease.

Because of the language barrier, social isolation, and cultural shock, older Sikhs also have an increased risk of depression.

Because Sikhs refrain from smoking, they tend to have lower rates of diseases closely associated with smoking. Sikh women also have lower rates of breast cancer.

Generally, Sikhs will also consult any medical professional in their extended family before making any major surgical decision.

Approaches to Decision Making

Most decisions are made collectively as a family, but families tend to rely on their physician to give an opinion. Generally, Sikhs will also consult any medical professional in their extended family before making any major surgical decision.

End-of-Life Care

In matters of terminal care, the attending physician should consult the patient, the family, an ethicist, and preferably a Sikh scholar before making a final decision.

Health care providers, including physicians, nurses, and chaplains, should comfort terminally ill patients, making sure they are pain free, have their relatives and friends nearby, and have access to a Sikh *Granthi* who can recite *Gurbani* (writings of the Gurus) and perform

Sikh prayers. When their loved ones pass on, Sikhs console themselves with the recitation of their sacred hymns.

Cremation is traditional in Sikhism. Funeral and cremation arrangements should be made in advance in consultation with the family and according to the wishes of the dying or deceased patient, if possible. The body should be taken with minimal delay to the funeral home for expeditious cremation, unless the family is waiting for a close relative to arrive. Routine post-mortem care should be provided, and the body covered with clean linens and shrouded. If the person is wearing any of the five Ks, they should remain with the body.

Cremation is traditional in Sikhism.

The family and Sikh *Granthi* should be allowed to follow Sikh traditions for preparing the body for funeral. The body should be treated with the same respect as during life. After cremation, prayers are said and food is served. If the patient was in hospice care, the family may wash and clothe the body immediately after death.

Advance Directives

Generally, planning for end-of-life care is a foreign concept to older Sikhs. They may be reluctant to have these discussions; some still believe that talking about death will make it a reality. Being tactful, taking time, and involving family members may make these discussions more palatable. Recommendations include identifying Sikh physicians or other health care providers on the staff who can act as liaisons with Sikh patients, informing individuals of their rights as patients, and encouraging patients to have advance directives.

Organ Donation and Transplantation

While there are some misgivings related to mutilation and reincarnation, and anxieties about technical or clinical aspects of the transplantation process, the prevailing Sikh view is supportive of transplantation. Organ donation is considered a highly appropriate means of exhibiting the altruistic tradition within Sikhism. Barriers surrounding transplantation seem to have more to do with knowledge and understanding than with cultural or religious factors.

Organ donation is considered a highly appropriate means of exhibiting the altruistic tradition within Sikhism.

CASE STUDY 1	**Cooperating with Sikh Family Members to Observe Religious Customs**

Objective

1. Understand the importance of religious symbols during minor surgical procedures.

You are an emergency room physician working on a weekend in a community hospital. An ambulance arrives with an older man. The EMT tells you that the man fell on the road and is bleeding from the scalp. When you see the patient, you determine that to have a clear field of vision, the hair in that area must be cut. While you are getting ready to tell the nurse to do so, the family arrives, and you discuss the case with them. They tell you that cutting the hair is prohibited and ask you for other options to control the bleeding. Followers of Sikhism believe that hair is a gift from God and that hair should not be cut or trimmed.

Finally, it is decided that because the bleeding is not that severe, it may be controlled by applying pressure to the scalp area, although it may be more time-consuming. Family members are willing to hold the pressure dressing, and the bleeding stops. The patient and the family are very appreciative of the understanding shown by the emergency room staff.

CASE STUDY 2 | When There Is No Advance Directive

Objectives

1. Many patients do not like to take their medicines for silent diseases, especially when they are told that such treatment may be lifelong.
2. Understand the importance of quality of life in Sikhism.

Mrs. Shaan is 71 years old. Her husband, Mr. Jasbir Singh, is 74 years old and in fairly good health. Their two children are first-generation immigrants to the United States. The oldest son is a doctor, and the younger one is a software engineer. The family members are religious and get their support from the God.

Mrs. Shaan has a history of hypertension for which she takes medication but not properly. She takes the medication only when she has a headache, believing that she will become addicted to it and that unless she is having a problem, there is no need for it. The doctor son has tried explaining to her in detail the need to take her antihypertensive medication regularly. She agrees with him but goes back to her own style after a few days. Her husband supports her.

While watching television, she gets a severe headache that she ignores for a while. Then her speech starts to slur, and she develops one-sided weakness. The Shaans call their son, and he advises them to call an ambulance immediately; he meets them in the emergency room. A CT scan shows a very big infarct. Mrs. Shaan is unresponsive and put on ventilator support. In the first few days, her family thinks she is responding to stimuli and opening her eyes and recognizing them. Several attempts made to wean her off the ventilator are unsuccessful. Finally, a tracheostomy is done, and a feeding tube is inserted. After a few days, Mrs. Shaan is transferred to a nursing home on a ventilator. She tries to move a hand and tries several times to say something, but after a few days she is no longer doing any of these. The family decides that Mrs. Shaan no longer has any quality of life. In absence of an advance directive, value systems are discussed, and it is decided to remove the life support. The husband expresses a desire to call organ donation, for which Mrs. Shaan is assessed. Hymns are read, and everybody prays around her. The life support is removed and, after a few hours, Mrs. Shaan passes away peacefully. Her husband is sad but understands that he did what she would have wanted if she were able to talk. He thanks the Almighty Lord for the time they had together.

Discussion Points:

- Advance directives should be done while in good health. It prevents undue suffering and saves loved ones from feeling guilty for making certain decisions.
- Sikhism values quality of life and honors the wishes of the patient and the family, who decide together.
- Sikhism is not averse to organ donation.
- Followers of Sikhism believe that everything happens in His will, and their prayer is always to receive the strength to accept it.

Upinder Singh, MD

References

Dhillon KS. *Functions, Duties, and Qualifications of a Granthi.* Available at: www.gurunanakdarbar.net/1DutiesandFunctionsofaGranthi.pdf (accessed November 2007).

What is Sikhism? Available at: http://www.gurunanakdarbar.net/New_Articles.htm (accessed November 2007).

Additional Resources

http://religiousmovements.lib.virginia.edu/nrms/sikhs.html

Shiromani Gurdwara Parbandhak Committee. The code of Sikh conduct and conventions. Amritsar, India. Council for a Parliament of the World's Religions, Chicago (tel: 312-629-2990).

Sikh American Heritage Organization
   tel: 630-377-5893

Sikh Religious Society of Chicago
   tel: 847-358-1117 or 847-359-5142

www.gurunanakdarbar.net

www.sikhnet.com

www.sikhs.org

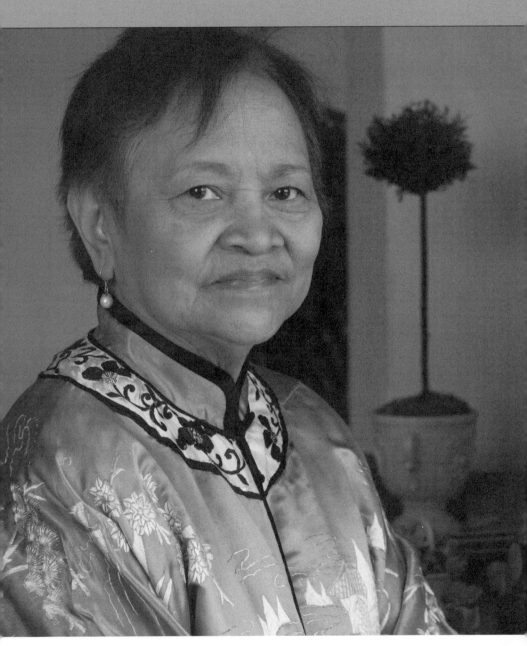

CHAPTER 10

Confucianism and Daoism

History

The teaching of Confucianism, as inherited and communicated by Confucius (551–479 BCE), is steeped in the concept of the *Dao*—the Way of Morality and Virtue—and the transcendental *Tian* (heaven). Thus for the Confucians, living a virtuous and moral life amounts to a perpetual prayer, the way to the Transcendent, and a path toward self-transcendence.

For the Confucians, living a virtuous and moral life amounts to a perpetual prayer.

The origin of Confucianism is lost in the mist of antiquity. Even so, it is safe to state that it predates Christianity by more than a millennium. Some scholars have traced its development to the Shang court, which worshiped the *Ti* (the Supreme Being) or *Shangti* (the Lord-on-High), who might have been the primogenitor of the Shang dynasty, traditionally dated from BCE 16th to the 11th centuries. Some scholars also argue that *Tian, Ti,* and *Shangti* could very well be one and the same deity who was called different names by people from various regions. The form of Confucianism we have today is the result of the long centuries of evolution shaped by scholars of the Han (BCE 206–220 CE), the Song (960–1279 CE), and the Ming (1368–1644 CE) dynasties.

The origin of Daoism, like its Confucian counterpart, is likewise difficult to determine. However, scholars generally divide Daoism into philosophical and religious camps, with the philosophical school beginning possibly as early as the sixth century BCE, while the second century CE saw the rise and establishment of religious Daoism, which probably had its origin in the ancient shamanism of the Shang dynasty.

Like their Confucian counterparts, the philosophical Daoists also view the *Dao*—the Way of Nature—as the most important principle. Therefore, living in accordance with this principle or the Way is of primary concern.

The philosophical Daoists also view the Dao—the Way of Nature—as the most important principle.

What then is the difference between Confucianism's and philosophical Daoism's understanding of the *Dao*? The difference lies in each tradition's emphasis: Confucianism emphasizes the importance of human relations, while philosophical Daoism stresses the importance of human relations with Nature.

Religious Daoism is pantheistic, monastic, and ritualistic.

Religious Daoism, on the other hand, is pantheistic, monastic, and ritualistic, with countless numbers of divine beings in the pantheon and a good number of rituals to adhere to. The Jade Emperor is considered to be the highest divine being. However, monasteries and temples are at liberty to choose to worship different deities altogether.

Important Holidays and Celebrations

Five important lunar seasonal festivals/holidays are shared by the Confucians and the Daoists—in fact by all Chinese: the Lunar New Year (*chunjie*), which normally falls between January 15 and February 18 in the solar calendar; the Clear and Bright (*qingming*), usually in April; the Dragon Boat Festival (*duanwu*), between May 15 and June 15; the Mid-autumn or Moon (*zhongqiu*) Festival, in early September; and the Double Yang (*chongyang*), late September to October 15.

During the Clear and Bright and Double Yang festivals, the Chinese (with some exceptions) go to the cemeteries to clear the graves of the ancestors and to make sacrifices to them.

In addition to these shared festivals, the Confucian tradition has designated September 28 (Confucius' birthday) in the solar calendar as Teachers Day, and the Daoists have designated the 15th day of the seventh moon or the first full moon of autumn as the *Zhongyuan* (Middle Primordial) Festival. Both are important in their own right. The Confucians celebrate Teachers Day in honor of educators (Confucius was considered the first private teacher of China), while the Daoist *Zhongyuan* is a festival of ancestral offerings.

Sacred Objects and Scriptures

Confucianism takes the secular as the sacred.

Confucianism takes the secular as the sacred. In fact, in Confucian thought, the two realms are not distinct. Therefore, identifying particular objects that would/could be considered sacred in this tradition is difficult. Yet we can say that high places—hills and mountains—because of their traditional association with religions, are often viewed as sacred. Ancestral spirit places and ancestral temples could also belong to the realm of the sacred. In both Confucianism and Daoism, the homes are sacred, because they are also temples in which most of the rituals are performed.

In religious Daoism, space is sacred because both divine beings and human beings occupy it. The diagram of the Great Ultimate (*taiji tu*), where Dao resides, is a sacred object in every temple. As with its Confucian counterpart, spirit places, occupied by both ancestral spirits and divine beings, are sacred. The sword, the talisman (*fu*), the bowl of water, and the horn are some of the sacred paraphernalia in the Daoist rituals, especially in the ritual for healing the sick.

Both Confucianism and Daoism are scriptural religions. The Confucian Canon consists of nine books; the Daoist Canon comprises thousands of texts. Unlike the Confucian Canon, the Daoist Canon is studied only by religious professionals. On the other hand, some hold the view that the Confucian Canon occupies a position in Chinese culture comparable to that occupied in the West by the Bible plus the major works of Greek and Roman literature.

Diverse Subgroups

From the Song dynasty until the 19th century, two major Confucian schools—the School of Principle and the School of Heart/Mind—were dedicated to carrying on the tradition. Since the 20th century, another school—the School of Contemporary New Confucians—has been added to the list of Confucian subgroups. In reality, this late-comer continues the teachings of the traditional schools, except that the scholars of this school tend to make use of Western philosophical tools in interpreting the Confucian principles.

Two prominent religious Daoist subgroups, both present in America, carry on the teachings of Daoism: the Heavenly Master School, a more ritualistically oriented southern group, and the Perfect Truth School, a more monastically oriented northern group. The former claims to continue the tradition of the first Daoist master, while the latter was organized during the Song dynasty and incorporated many teachings from both Confucianism and Buddhism into its doctrines and practices.

Both Confucianism and Daoism have shaped the hearts and minds of the Chinese people inside China proper, as well as within the Chinese cultural universe. In addition, nations such as Japan, Korea,

Confucianism and Daoism have shaped the hearts and minds of the Chinese people inside China proper, as well as within the Chinese cultural universe.

Vietnam, and Singapore have been heavily influenced by Confucianism and Daoism. The government of Indonesia recognizes Confucianism as one of the national religions.

Even so, the vast majority of the Chinese today would not identify themselves as Confucians. They simply live the Confucian Way of life—a life of morality, virtue, and mutual obligations, without feeling the need for self-identification with Confucianism or acknowledging acceptance of Confucian orthodoxy. And, in general, the Chinese from within China proper are less inclined to identify with religions than the Chinese from other areas.

Terms and Roles for Spiritual Leaders and Advisors

"Pastoral care," a term associated with Western Christianity, may have no meaning to a person who is not Christian. In traditional China, family members, doctors, or Daoist priests care for the sick.

Religious Basis for Views on Health and Disease

The development of traditional Chinese medicine was based on the theories of *yin* and *yang* and the five elements: metal (*jin*), wood (*mu*),

Diseases are considered to be the imbalance of the yin *and* yang *and the five elements.*

water (*shui*), fire (*huo*), and earth (*tu*). To have good health is to maintain a proper balance among these five elements. Diseases are considered to be the imbalance of the *yin* and *yang* and the five elements. Sometimes, it is also stated that disease is due to the imbalance of *qi*, which has two basic meanings. First, it is the "stuff" along with the Great Ultimate that gives birth to everything in the cosmos; second, it is the "stuff" in each one of us, but it needs to be cultivated/nourished or *yangqi*. Confucians usually follow the traditional understanding of *yin, yang,* and *qi*.

Religious Daoists consider "sin" or "ghosts" to be the cause of illness.

Religious Daoists, on the other hand, consider "sin" or "ghosts" to be the cause of illness.

This, however, is not to say that both Confucianism and Daoism reject the modern views of health and disease. In fact, older generation Chinese often embrace both Chinese traditional and Western medical practices. Older Chinese adults have a high degree of respect for Western-trained physicians, and they are often pleased when their physicians take the time to explain their medical conditions or to ask their wishes on treatment options. In matters of serious illness or impending death, physicians are often reluctant to engage in difficult discussions with Chinese patients, often citing the misconception that discussions of death are cultural taboo for older Chinese people.

Older generation Chinese often embrace both Chinese traditional and Western medical practices.

Dietary Restrictions

All properties of food are classified as *yin* or *yang*, ie, cold or hot, although this has nothing to do with the actual temperature of the food. It has everything to do with seeking balance in the foods we eat.

Traditionally, dietary restrictions are not imposed on older adults. In fact, older adults are often allowed to eat what they like, with respect to the realization that the end of life is in sight and they should have the food they enjoy. However, some contemporary Chinese older adults do observe dietary restrictions under the order of a doctor or a nutritionist.

Traditionally, dietary restrictions are not imposed on older adults.

Gender Considerations

Confucianism maintains that human nature is good. This goodness, bestowed by Tian (heaven) is found in every human being. Thus, from an ontological perspective, there is gender equality in Confucianism. The Confucian society, however, is hierarchical in structure. Even so, it can be argued that in function, there is social equality between the sexes, because all human relations are governed by the principle of reciprocity.

Religious Daoism has treated both sexes far more equally, at least in religious matters. From the beginning, religious Daoism had and still has both male and female libationers—priests and priestesses—performing the same religious and ritual functions on an equal basis.

Still, it would be quite blind not to acknowledge that male Confucians and Daoists, as in every society dominated by men, have not been very kind to the opposite sex. Chinese society continues today to value men more than women.

Beliefs about Death and Life after Death

Confucians believe that life and death constitute a continuum. The living depend on the dead for advice and guidance in daily matters,

Confucians believe that life and death constitute a continuum.

and the dead rely on the living for sustenance. Confucians also believe that each individual has two souls—the *hun* soul, which ascends to heaven when the person dies, and the *po* soul, which remains with the corpse.

Even though Confucians value life and would do everything possible to preserve it (because it is given by the parents), they would not hesitate to condone suicide in some situations if by doing so the individual would achieve a higher principle of virtue/morality for the sake of the greater good. Furthermore, euthanasia and abandonment, voluntary or otherwise, of older adults was also practiced in ancient China.

Modern China has no official policies on euthanasia and abandonment. Suicides do occur but without official sanction or condemnation.

In philosophical Daoism, ie, in the *Zhuang Zi,* death is generally presented and considered as a natural phenomenon that need neither

In philosophical Daoism, death is generally presented and considered as a natural phenomenon.

be feared nor desired but that can be accepted as it comes. There is also a story in the same book about the death of Zhuang Zi's wife, in which Zhuang Zi seems to maintain that the dead are better off than the living.

In religious Daoism, death is a big sickness or a total disorder.

In religious Daoism, death is a big sickness or a total disorder. It is conceived as the dispersal of *qi*. In addition, religious Daoists believe in the existence of both heaven and hell, as well as in human souls. If a dead person had the misfortune to end up in hell, that person invariably would be tormented by the beings of the underworld.

The Daoist hell is more akin to the Catholic idea of purgatory rather than a permanent place without any possibility of redemption for the condemned.

Even though both traditions believe in heaven and hell, they have little to say about heaven. And the Daoists have much more to say about hell than the Confucians.

Healing and Health-Promoting Ceremonies and Rituals

Confucians since the Song dynasty have considered capping (a rite of passage for boys), wedding, funeral, and sacrificial rites as the four major family rituals—which may or may not have anything to do with healing and health-promoting ceremonies and rituals. However, Confucianism does stress the ideas of "quiet sitting" (*jingzuo*) and the elimination of "desire" (*yu*) as a means of spiritual exercise and self-cultivation. It could arguably be claimed that this might be a Confucian way toward developing good personal health. After all, the practice of "quiet sitting" and the elimination of "desire" can be done individually and involve no spiritual specialist.

> *Confucianism does stress the ideas of "quiet sitting" (jingzuo) and the elimination of "desire" (yu) as a means of spiritual exercise and self-cultivation.*

Religious Daoism definitely has a healing and health-promoting ritual. Illness is considered a "disorder" (*luan*), caused by "sin" (*zui*) or a "ghost" (*gui*). To heal the sick is to "govern" (*zhi*) the "disorder" by means of an exorcism ritual involving the use of a talisman (which represents the order of a divine being), a bowl of water, and a sword. This ritual is performed in front of the altar in a Daoist temple by the priest or the priestess. After the ritual is over, the talisman is burnt and the ashes are mixed in with the water. The water has now become talisman-water to be drunk by the sick person. Daoist rituals, in addition to being religious, also have a therapeutic aspect in reorienting one's perception of the world order and in providing temporary relief in the daily life of an individual.

> *Daoist rituals also have a therapeutic aspect in reorienting one's perception of the world order.*

Views on Do-Not-Resuscitate Orders, Nutrition, and Hydration at the End of Life

Older Chinese adults, especially first-generation US immigrants, are reluctant to speak about death, believing that just talking about it can bring bad omens. Many older adults believe that there is a natural time for death, that death at an old age is expected. The desire is for a natural, peaceful death. Some have used the metaphor of the long road coming to an end. For most who have led a full life and who have supportive family, death is not feared.

> *Older Chinese adults are reluctant to speak about death.*

Few older Chinese adults sign legal documents such as Durable Powers of Attorneys for Health Care to express advance directives. There are two, possibly three, influential factors. First, many older Chinese immigrants have limited English literacy skills, and the accepted

Many older Chinese immigrants have limited English literacy skills.

legal instruments are in English. Second, the reluctance to sign legal documents reflects the cultural importance the Chinese place on the honor of the spoken word and verbal agreements. A third factor could be that the act of signing a document may be considered acknowledgement of the end and, thus, may be considered an omen.

It is important for physicians caring for older Chinese adults to engage the patient in meaningful discussions of advance directives and then to accept the verbal decisions as binding. The two most important issues that physicians should discuss are whether to initiate cardiopulmonary resuscitation in the event of natural cardiac arrest (death), and whether to provide nutrition and hydration through enteral feeding tubes if the patient can no longer drink fluids or take oral feedings. At On Lok Senior Health Services in San Francisco, which serves more than 600 frail Chinese adults, more than 90% of the Chinese adults choose do-not-resuscitate and an equal percentage choose not to have feeding tubes if they could not eat naturally. "When my time comes, let me go naturally and peacefully."

In Chinese culture, decision making is not individual but leans on the wishes of the extended family.

The physician should be aware of cultural factors relevant to the patient's decision making. In Chinese culture, decision making is not individual but leans on the wishes of the extended family. Very often, older adults defer major decisions for their own health to their children, particularly sons. Sometimes, this deference to children for major health care decisions results in conflicts if the patient's wishes are not known. If an older Chinese adult has made known a preference for no life-sustaining treatment, the children will comply out of filial obligation. Otherwise, the children may choose to continue heroic and sometimes futile measures, out of a sense of filial obligation to maintain life to the utmost.

Religious Customs and Rituals for Dying Patients and After Death

The religious ritual for the dying in Confucianism is part of elaborate funeral rites. In traditional China, before hospitals were introduced, people typically died in family homes. In preparation for death, the dying person was moved to the main room of the house. Once the person died, a soul-calling ceremony was performed. In modern society, this ritual is seldom performed. Even though there is a standard and formal funeral rite for the dead, families seldom perform it in its entirety. It is both too lengthy and too costly. Both traditional and modern families often choose elements from it for the funeral. In today's China, the preferred method of disposing of the body is cremation. As stated above, the fourth ritual in Confucianism is the sacrificial rite to the ancestors. This ritual, in its much-modified form, continues to be performed for the dead annually during the Bright and Clear and the Double Yang festivals.

In today's China, the preferred method of disposing of the body is cremation.

Religious Daoism also calls for a very elaborate funeral ritual. It consists of four parts: the soul-calling (*zhaohun*), the opening of the path of dark hell (*kaiming lu*), the crossing of the bridge (*guoqiao*), and the burning of the storehouse money (*shaoku qian*). The aim of the funeral ritual is exorcistic, ie, to get rid of the dead.

Religious Daoism also calls for a very elaborate funeral ritual.

Some time after the funeral, members of the family may request a soul-releasing (*chaodu*) ritual be performed to release the soul of the dead from suffering. And like their Confucian counterparts, the Daoists also observe sacrificial rites for their ancestors.

In Confucianism, the members of the family conduct the rituals, whereas in Daoism, the priests and priestesses do so.

| CASE STUDY 1 | Suicide or Cultural Norm?: The Case of an Older Chinese Adult |

Objectives
1. Consider the cultural context of an older Chinese adult who refuses food and hydration near the end of life. Does it conform to the acceptance of a natural and peaceful end of life?
2. Discuss the appropriateness of applying mental health concepts such as depression and suicide when treating older Chinese patients near the end of life.

A 92-year-old Chinese man with major depressive disorder began to actively refuse food and hydration, stating he wished to die. He had previously expressed wishes for no aggressive or life-prolonging treatments, including placement of a feeding tube.

He was born in a southern province of China as the only son of three children in a family of farmers. He reared three children, two sons and a daughter, while establishing a successful business in Vietnam. He was widowed at age 69 and immigrated to the United States at age 75 to live with one of his sons. His oldest son died unexpectedly when the patient was 82 years old.

The patient was in good health and physically active until the last 4 years, during which he became more frail and was not able to walk in the community without help. His daughter-in-law provided most of his care at home. On many occasions, the patient expressed sadness over his loss of independence. About 2 months before death, he began to refuse food and hydration, despite coaxing from his family.

Question:
1. Was the patient's behavior in the final months of life consistent with his cultural values of self and family?

Mental health professionals who evaluated him agreed that he was expressing the equivalent of suicidal intent and placed him in a psychiatric facility (under 5150 authority) to prevent further self-harm. He remained hospitalized for 28 days, making very little progress. Despite treatment with antidepressants and the long hospitalization, he did not regain weight and continued to demonstrate willful self-deprivation of food and hydration.

Questions:

1. In Western mental health practice, depression is treatable and suicide is considered preventable if treatment is timely. In this case, was the patient demonstrating cultural acceptance of aging and losses, or was this a depressive illness that required treatment?
2. Was the death from natural causes, or was it a result of failed treatment for depression?

The clinicians faced the dilemma of how to treat this frail patient. Aggressive intervention would require insertion of a feeding tube against his wishes. Ethics consultation was sought. The Ethics Committee advised respecting the patient's wishes and providing him with a palliative care plan while continuing his antidepressants. The man died peacefully 8 days later in the presence of family.

Questions:

1. What was the significance of continuing antidepressants in the palliative plan?
2. Were the patient's verbally expressed advance directives for health care, made years before his final illness, adequate in this case?

| CASE STUDY **2** | **The Interplay of Tradition, Perception, Values, and Faith** |

Objectives

1. Discuss how religious diversity and cultural values may help treatment decisions.
2. Review the cultural/religious/perceptual basis for Mrs. Wu's request to help her "leave this world" in dignity and peace.
3. Discuss how your understanding of your own ethics may or may not help you in honoring Mrs. Wu's request.

In 1997, Mrs. Wu, age 65, emigrated from Taiwan to join her son in the United States. Initially, she did not want to come to America, because she had friends and family in Taiwan. But having been brought up in a traditional family, which upholds harmony as a highly desirable virtue, Mrs. Wu along with her unmarried daughter reluctantly yielded to Mr. Wu's decision to come.

Mrs. Wu is a high school graduate. Her husband, who was a teacher in Taiwan, is presently retired with limited income. He is quite well educated in Confucian thoughts and practices and is no stranger to philosophical Daoism. The son, a graduate of an American university, has a lackadaisical attitude toward organized religions but claims to be spiritual. The daughter, also a university graduate, is a faithful follower of religious Daoism and values both Confucian teachings and Daoist practices.

Recently, Mrs. Wu began to complain about having heartburn sensations, especially after each meal. At first, the family decided to get some Chinese traditional medicine to restore the imbalance in her body. But that did not seem to work. The daughter suggested that the family engage a Daoist priest to perform some healing rituals for her mother. Her brother was very much opposed to the idea and thought his mother should see a Western physician instead. Mr. Wu was reluctant to follow the advice of his adult children, which was compounded by his conviction that people must face their mortality and accept whatever comes their way with equanimity.

Mrs. Wu, caught between her adult children's desire to help and her husband's reluctance to follow the children's advice, decided not to seek treatment. Several months went by, and Mrs. Wu's discomfort continued. Mr. Wu reluctantly sided with his son.

After listening to Mrs. Wu's description of her symptoms, you told the family that you suspected Mrs. Wu was suffering from an acid condition. You suggested that an endoscopy of the upper gastrointestinal tract be performed to assess the situation more fully. The son thought it was a good idea, but Mr. Wu was concerned about the cost. The daughter maintained that such a procedure, if performed at all, should be done in the presence of a Daoist priest. Sensing her husband's concern, Mrs. Wu was unwilling to undergo the procedure.

Six months later, the family returned to your office with a Daoist priest in tow. The family now agreed to the endoscopy procedure, providing that the priest was allowed to be present.

Questions:
1. What are the advantages or disadvantages of allowing the priest to be present in the procedure room?
2. If you decide not to admit the priest, how would you explain your decision without giving the family the impression that you have violated "their culture"?

The procedure and subsequent biopsy confirmed that Mrs. Wu had cancer of the esophagus. You suggest surgery to prolong—and possibly save—her life. Mrs. Wu immediately rejected your suggestion, because to her an operation involved "cutting up" the body, where the *po* soul would reside after her death.

Questions:
1. How would you respond to Mrs. Wu's rejection without making her feel that you are being disrespectful of her tradition?
2. When Mrs. Wu contrasts your wisdom, knowledge, and authority with her humble station, what was really going on in her mind?

Her son became angry with his mother's seeming ignorance of modern sciences and her holding onto those "old ideas," while her daughter insisted that her mother would be all right through the performance of the Daoist healing rituals. Finally, Mrs. Wu asked to speak with you in private. She acknowledged her respect for your medical wisdom, knowledge, and authority as well as her humble station in life. At the end of the conversation, she begged you to help her "leave this world" with dignity and peace.

Questions:
1. How would you handle Mrs. Wu's request on the basis of her culture?

2. What are the ethical issues that need to be considered from your perspective and from Mrs. Wu's?

This case study brings out the conflicting perspectives within the wide spectrum of belief and non-belief that may exist within immigrant families. The physician may need training in how to mediate between these widely differing perspectives among key family members, as well as in dealing with the possible presence of indigenous spiritual care leaders, a practice with which the physician may not be familiar.

Edmond Yee, PhD
Catherine Eng, MD

References

Berger JT. Commentary: culture and ethnicity in clinical care. *Arch Intern Med* 1998;158:2085–2090.

Eleazer GP, Hornung CA, Egbert CB, et al. The relationship between ethnicity and advance directives in a frail elderly population. *J Am Geriatr Soc* 1996;44:938–943.

Hsi C. *Chu Hsi's Family Rituals*. Princeton, NJ: Princeton University Press; 1991 (trans. PB Ebrey).

Lagerwey J. *Taoist Ritual in Chinese Society and History*. New York: Macmillan Publishing Company; 1987.

McLaughlin LA, Braun KL. Asian and Pacific Islander cultural values: considerations for health care decision making. *Health Social Work* 1998;23(2):116–126.

Thompson LG. *Chinese Religion: An Introduction* (3rd ed). Belmont, CA: Wadsworth, Inc; 1979.

Tu W, Tucker ME (eds). *Confucian Spirituality*. New York: Crossroad Publishing Company; 2003.

Wong E. *The Shambhala Guide to Taoism*. Boston: Shambhala; 1997.

Yao X. *An Introduction to Confucianism*. Cambridge, England: Cambridge University Press; 2000.

INDEX

This index covers Volumes I, II, and III of Doorway Thoughts. The page numbers are preceded by "I", "II", or "III" to indicate in which volume the topic appears.

A

Ablution, Islamic, III:86
Acculturation
  of American Indian and Alaska Native elders, I:19
  of Asian Indian American elders, I:71
  of Buddhists, III:23
  of Cambodian American elders, II:40–II:41
  case studies, I:103–I:104, II:89–II:90
  of Chinese American elders, I:97, I:103–I:104
  of Filipino American elders, II:61–II:62
  of Haitian American elders, II:79, II:89–II:90
  health beliefs and behavior and, I:7, II:7–II:8
  of Hindus, III:63–III:64
  of Hispanic American elders, I:30–I:31
  of Japanese American elders, I:83
  of Korean American elders, II:99
  of Muslims, III:86
  of Pakistani American elders, II:117
  of Portuguese American elders, II:138–II:139
  of Russian-speaking American elders, II:155
  of Vietnamese American elders, I:57
Addressing patients, I:4, II:4
Adler, Reva N., I:3–I:15, II:2–II:14
Advance directives, use of, I:11–I:12, II:13–II:14
  by African American elders, I:47
  by American Indian and Alaska Native elders, I:22
  by Asian Indian American elders, I:75
  by Buddhist American elders, III:29
  by Cambodian American elders, II:48
  case studies, I:64–I:67
  by Chinese American elders, I:101–I:102, III:153
  by Filipino American elders, II:68
  by Haitian American elders, II:87–II:88
  by Hindu American elders, III:68
  by Hispanic American elders, I:35–I:36

  by Japanese American elders, I:86
  by Korean American elders, II:104–II:105
  by Muslim American elders, III:88–III:89
  by Portuguese American elders, II:143
  by Russian-speaking American elders, II:159
  by Sikh American elders, III:141, III:143–III:144
  by Vietnamese American elders, I:60
Advent, Christian seasons, III:43
African American elders, I:43–I:53
  approaches to decision making, I:46
  case studies, I:48–I:53
  disclosure and consent for, I:46–I:47
  doorway thoughts for, I:43
  end-of-life decision making and care intensity, I:47
  formality of address, I:43
  gender issues, I:47
  health risks, I:45–I:46
  immigration status, I:45
  language and literacy, I:43–I:44
  preferred cultural terms, I:43
  respectful nonverbal communication with, I:44
  tradition and health beliefs, I:45
  use of advance directives, I:47
  use of North American health services by, I:44
African American (term), I:39
African Methodist Episcopal denomination, III:42
After death care
  Buddhist, III:26–III:27
  Christian, III:50–III:51
  Confucian and Daoist, III:154–III:155
  Hindu, III:69
  Hmong, III:128
  Jewish, III:109
  Sikh, III:141
Afterlife, Buddhism and, III:25–III:26
Ahimsa, in Buddhist belief, III:29
Alaska Native (term), I:17
Alaska Natives. *see* American Indian and Alaska Native elders

163

of Haitian American elders, II:80
of Hindus, III:63
of Hispanic American elders, I:30
of Hmong, III:120–III:121
of Japanese American elders, I:82–I:83
of Korean American elders, II:98–II:99
of Pakistani American elders, II:116
of Portuguese American elders,
    II:137–II:138
of Russian-speaking American elders,
    II:154–II:155
of Vietnamese American elders, I:57
Incense, healing rituals and, III:127
Indian (term), I:17, I:69
Indian Health Service (IHS), I:20
Indians
    American. *see* American Indian and Alaska
        Native elders
    Asian. *see* Asian Indian American elders
Informed consent, I:9–I:10. *see also* Disclosure
    and consent
Interpreters
    case study, I:64–I:67
    need for, I:4
Iraqi American (term), II:21
Iraqi Americans. *see* Arab American elders
Islam. *see also* Pakistani American elders
    advance directives, III:88–III:89
    Arab American elders. *see* Arab American
        elders
    barriers to quality health care, III:86
    beliefs regarding illness, III:87
    case studies, III:91–III:94
    cultural and religious practices affecting
        health care, III:84
    death and dying beliefs, III:90
    dietary practices, III:85
    disclosure and consent regarding health
        crises, III:88
    diversity among Muslims, III:81
    end-of-life care, III:88
    gender issues, III:84
    holidays and celebrations, III:82
    holy texts, III:82
    Muslim family structure, III:83–III:84
    overview, III:81
    palliative care beliefs, III:89
    religious basis for views on health and
        illness, III:82–III:83
    rituals affecting health care, III:85–III:86
    spiritual advisers in health care setting,
        III:87
Issei (first-generation Japanese Americans),
    I:83

J

Japanese American elders, I:81–I:93
    acculturation, I:83

approaches to decision making, I:85
case studies, I:87–I:92
disclosure and consent for, I:85
doorway thoughts for, I:81
end-of-life decision making and care
    intensity, I:85–I:86, I:87–I:89, I:90–I:93
formality of address, I:81–I:82
gender issues, I:85
health risks, I:84
immigration history, I:82–I:83
language and literacy, I:82
preferred cultural terms, I:81
respectful nonverbal communication with,
    I:82
tradition and health beliefs, I:83–I:84
use of advance directives, I:86
Japanese Americans, Buddhism and, III:27–
    III:28
Japanese Americans (term), I:81
Jesus Christ, III:38–III:39
Jingzuo (quiet sitting), Confucianism, III:153
Joint Commission on Accreditation of
    Healthcare Organizations, III:3
Judaism
    case studies, III:110–III:114
    Christianity and, III:38
    death and dying beliefs, III:107–III:109
    dietary practices, III:105
    end-of-life care, III:107–III:108
    gender issues, III:105–III:106
    healing ceremonies and rituals, III:106
    history of, III:99–III:100
    holidays and celebrations, III:100–III:102
    overview, III:99
    religious beliefs regarding health and
        disease, III:104–III:105
    sacred objects and scriptures, III:102–
        III:103
    spiritual adviser role in health care,
        III:103–III:104
    subgroups, III:103

K

Kairos, III:48
Karma
    Buddhist beliefs, III:24–III:25
    Hindu beliefs, I:72, III:61–III:62
Keo, Yani Rose, II:37–II:48
Khalsa, Sikh symbols, III:135–III:136
Khatutsky, Galina, II:153–II:160
Khmer, II:37. *see also* Cambodian American
    elders
Khmer Loeu, II:37. *see also* Cambodian
    American elders
Khsaoy beh daung ("weak heart" syndrome),
    II:44
Khyol (wind illness), II:41–II:42
Kibbei, I:83

Sohn, Linda, II:97–II:105
Song dynasty, III:147
Southeast Asian American elders, II:37
Spirit helpers, Hmong, III:124
Spirits, Hmong, III:122
Spiritual advisers
    American Indians, III:13–III:14
    Buddhist, III:30
    Christian, III:44–III:45
    Confucian and Daoist, III:150
    help in decision-making, III:5
    incorporating into health care team, III:6
    Jewish, III:103–III:104
    Muslim, III:87
Spiritual history, in approach to patients,
    III:4–III:5
Spirituality
    case studies, I:37–I:38, II:30–II:31
    effect on health, III:4
    relationship to physical health in First
        Nations theology, III:12–III:13
    religion and, III:3
Stallworth, Monica, II:77–II:88
Suffering
    Christian beliefs, III:47
    Hindu beliefs, III:61
    Muslim beliefs, III:83
Suicide. see Euthanasia
Sukhāvatī, Pure Land Buddhism and, III:26
Sukkot, Jewish holidays, III:101
Sun Dance, III:10
Sunnah, III:82
Sunnis, III:81
Syrian American (term), II:21
Syrian Americans. see Arab American elders

T
Taboos, health care and, III:18
Taíno Indians, II:82
Talmud, III:103
Tanabe, Marianne K.G., I:81–I:93
Tanakh (Hebrew Bible), III:102
Terminal illness
    life-support technologies and, III:107–
        III:108
    Sikh beliefs, III:138
    spiritual support and, III:5
Terminology
    case study, II:144–II:146
    preferred cultural terms for African
        American elders, I:43
    preferred cultural terms for American
        Indian and Alaska Native elders, I:17
    preferred cultural terms for Arab American
        elders, II:21
    preferred cultural terms for Asian Indian
        American elders, I:69

    preferred cultural terms for Cambodian
        American elders, II:37
    preferred cultural terms for Chinese
        American elders, I:95
    preferred cultural terms for Filipino
        American elders, II:57–II:58
    preferred cultural terms for Haitian
        American elders, II:78
    preferred cultural terms for Hispanic
        American elders, I:29
    preferred cultural terms for Japanese
        American elders, I:81
    preferred cultural terms for Korean
        American elders, II:97
    preferred cultural terms for Pakistani
        American elders, II:113
    preferred cultural terms for Portuguese
        American elders, II:133
    preferred cultural terms for Russian-
        speaking American elders, II:153
    preferred cultural terms for Vietnamese
        American elders, I:55
    preferred terms for cultural identity,
        I:3–I:4, II:4
Theravāda Buddhism
    beliefs and doctrines, III:24–III:25
    Buddhism in America, III:23
    deathbed, mortuary, memorial rituals,
        III:26–III:2
    gender issues, III:28
    history of, III:24
    holidays and observances, III:26
Torah, III:102
Tradition and health beliefs, I:7–I:8, II:8–II:9
    of African American elders, I:45
    of American Indian and Alaska Native
        elders, I:19–I:20
    American Indians, III:9–III:10
    of Arab Americans, II:23–II:25,
        II:32–II:33
    of Asian Indian American elders, I:71–I:73
    barriers to quality health care, III:87
    of Buddhists, III:24–III:25
    of Cambodian American elders,
        II:41–II:42
    case studies, II:32–II:33, II:91–II:93,
        II:161–II:162
    of Chinese American elders, I:98–I:99,
        I:105–I:106
    of Christians, III:38–III:39
    of Confucians and Daoists, III:150–
        III:151
    of Filipino American elders, II:62–II:63
    of Haitian American elders, II:81–II:82,
        II:87, II:91–II:93
    health care and, III:6
    of Hindus, III:60–III:62, III:64–III:66
    of Hispanic American elders, I:31

CREDITS

American Geriatrics Society

The American Geriatrics Society (AGS) is a nationwide, not-for-profit association of geriatric health care professionals dedicated to improving the health, independence, and quality of life for all older people. The AGS promotes high quality, comprehensive, and accessible health care for America's older population, including those who are chronically ill and disabled. The Society provides leadership to health care professionals, policy makers, and the public by developing, implementing, and advocating programs in patient care, research, professional and public education, and public policy.

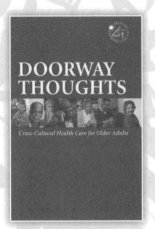
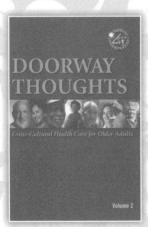

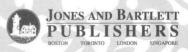